A SURGEON
IN THE VILLAGE

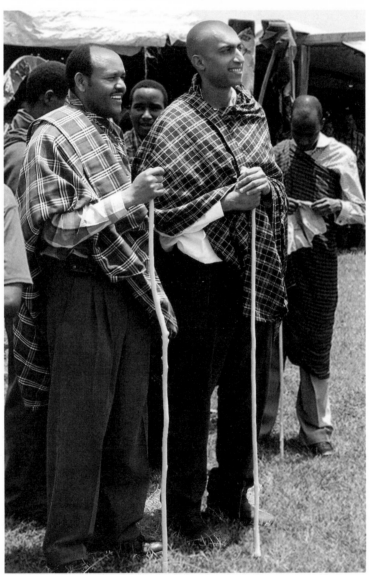

Emmanuel Mayegga of Tanzania stands with his friend and mentor from the United States, Dilan Ellegala, in Haydom, a remote town on the edge of Tanzania's Great Rift Valley. Photo by Liesbeth Hoek.

A SURGEON
in the VILLAGE

AN AMERICAN DOCTOR TEACHES
BRAIN SURGERY IN AFRICA

. . .

TONY BARTELME
with Catharina Hoek-Ellegala

Beacon Press
BOSTON

Beacon Press
Boston, Massachusetts
www.beacon.org

Beacon Press books
are published under the auspices of
the Unitarian Universalist Association of Congregations.

20 19 18 17   8 7 6 5 4 3 2 1

This book is printed on acid-free paper that meets the uncoated paper
ANSI/NISO specifications for permanence as revised in 1992.

Text design and composition by Kim Arney

Library of Congress Cataloging-in-Publication Data

Names: Bartelme, Tony. | Hoek-Ellegala, Catharina.
Title: A surgeon in the village : an American doctor teaches brain surgery
in Africa / Tony Bartelme ; with Catharina Hoek-Ellegala.
Other titles: Previous title: Send forth the healing sun
Description: Boston : Beacon Press, [2017] | Includes bibliographical references.
Identifiers: LCCN 2016030297| ISBN 9780807044889 (hardcover : alk. paper) |
ISBN 9780807044926 (e-book)
Subjects: LCSH: Ellegala, Dilantha B. | Neurosurgeons—United
States—Biography | Nervous system—Surgery—Tanzania. |
Medical care—Tanzania.
Classification: LCC RD592.9.E55 B37 2017 | DDC 617.4/8092 [B] —dc23
LC record available at https://lccn.loc.gov/2016030297

For Annie

CONTENTS

Language is fluid in Tanzania; many I met knew Swahili, English, and two local languages. And Sri Lanka presents its own special tongue twisters. So here's a pronunciation guide:

"Ohayoda" sounds like oh-hi-oooda.

Dilan's first name rhymes with Milan, and his last name is pronounced Ella-ghalla.

Mayegga is My-eh-guh.

Nuwas is New-ahs.

Hayte's first name is pronounced Hi-yeh-te.

Haydom is pronounced most often Hi-dom but also Hay-dom.

THE CALL

It's dry season in the Tanzanian bush, on a night when the stars pour across a blue-black sky. Suddenly the wind carries an unusual sound: "*Ohayoda! Ohayoda!*"

Maybe it's just a hyena—they hide on the hill below the hospital. No, there's urgency in this sound: it's someone crying out, "*Ohayoda! Ohayoda!*"

And it's not just one voice now. It's two, three, many; the night cries rise above the chorus of crickets, mosquitoes, and barking dogs. It's a wave, these voices, rising and breaking over the glass shards on the hospital wall. The wave flows through the screen windows of the guesthouse where the foreign doctors gather; it sweeps through the surgical wards, the children's ward, and then beyond, to the guard gates, the red dirt road to the airstrip, the *mamas* sitting by pans of sizzling eggs in Haydom town.

To a restaurant named Love.

You'll find Baba Naman, the hospital's radiologist, there on the restaurant's back stoop, watching the place he loves gather itself for the night. Emmanuel Mayegga, whom Naman loves like a son, often joins him for a beer, staring across time and distance to a space on the starlit horizon; wood smoke fills the air. "*Ohayoda!*"

Baba Naman explains: *Ohayoda* is a Datoga word, and it means "call to attention" and "call to action." If your child gets lost or your cow wanders off, then you stand outside your home and cry, "*Ohayoda!*" Naturally, your family and neighbors are curious about what's wrong. They leave their huts and *bomas* to find you. When they learn about your problem, they make it their own; they stand with you and shout with you. Word spreads quickly: hearing the call, a child may follow it home; a neighbor might spot the wandering cow.

Until the problem is solved, everyone stands together in the dark and shouts, "*Ohayoda! Ohayoda!*"

PART I

See One

Each time a man stands up for an ideal, or acts to improve the lot of others, or strikes out against injustice, he sends forth a tiny ripple of hope, and crossing each other from a million different centers of energy and daring, those ripples build a current which can sweep down the mightiest walls of oppression and resistance.

—SENATOR ROBERT F. KENNEDY,
to antiapartheid students in South Africa, 1966

Spread, suck, spread. Dilan Ellegala aimed the forceps deeper into the young woman's brain. Brain surgeons typically grab tissue with their forceps, but Dilan used the instrument in the opposite way: He kept the tips together to form a point; he pressed that point into her brain, pink and pulsing with her heart; then barely moving his hand, he released the pressure so the tips spread apart on their own. Doing this created a tiny space between the lobes. He suctioned fluid away with a long tube. *Perfect, now do it again, go deeper.*

He pressed his eyes to the lenses of the operating microscope. He worked the forceps as if by remote control. He did so in a rhythmic way, like a cat pawing at a rug. The trick was to find the right spot to place your tips. Miss that spot by just a fraction of a millimeter, and you could sever an artery. Miss that spot, and you might snuff out a lifetime of memories. But if your aim is true, you could peel apart someone's lobes like segments of an orange. You could go where other surgeons could not.

He'd learned this peeling technique from Arthur Day, his mentor here at Harvard Medical School and hands down the best neurosurgery teacher he ever had. Arthur Day was a brilliant technician when it came to microsurgery, but his true genius lay in how he forced you to question everything. Why did you move your forceps this way instead of that? Why did you choose this kind of aneurysm clip over another? Always why, until you realized that you truly didn't know everything about your patient's disease and how to fix it. But now, because of this revelation, you could learn more about the anatomy; you could plan a better strategy, move closer to the sun. "Perfection, that's what we're after," Arthur Day told you over and over, and then he fixed this knowledge into your brain by giving you a chance to soar or fuck up.

Like now. Dilan was just a few months into a vascular fellowship at Harvard's Brigham and Women's Hospital, but here he was doing a cardiac standstill, heart and brain surgery in one, climbing Mount Everest. *Awesome*, he'd thought earlier that morning as he scrubbed in. This was why he'd spent five years in medical school at the University of Washington. This was why he went through another eight years of research and residency, much of it at the University of Virginia, one of the toughest neurosurgery departments in the country. This was the ultimate final exam. One out of three standstill patients died on the table, in post-op, or while recuperating. As far as anyone knew at the Brigham, this was the first standstill ever done in New England. Maybe twenty people on the planet had the skills and balls to do a standstill. Twenty-four astronauts flew to the moon. Dilan thought, *I'm doing things that other doctors only read about.*

He didn't know much about the woman on the table. She was Arthur Day's patient. Dilan was the back-shop mechanic—the guy with grease on his hands, the one who rarely saw the customer.

One thing Dilan did know: this patient had run out of options. The human brain is soaked in blood—four hundred miles of vessels course through it. Under the beating pressure of the heart, some of this plumbing can weaken. In a particularly weak spot, the vessel develops a tiny aneurysm sac. Like an overfilled balloon, the vessel's wall gets thinner as it stretches—so thin you can see through it and watch blood swirl about. You never know when an aneurysm might burst: after a fall, a slap on the back, or simply standing up. Sex is a common trigger, which doctors call a coital headache. When an aneurysm ruptures, billions of neural networks suddenly go dark, like a city in a blackout. One out of ten people die instantaneously. Half of those who make it to the operating room end up dead within six months. Many survivors are brain-damaged for life.

The woman's aneurysm was huge, nearly an inch long. And it was next to the brain stem, which controlled heartbeat, breathing, and other critical functions. And feeding this control center were perforator vessels, some as thin as spiderweb strands. Cut just one strand, and you might sever a link from the brain to the heart. Your margin of error was zero. All in all, her aneurysm was in one of the most delicate, protected, and difficult-to-reach places in the human body. The only way to fix it was to build a tunnel through her brain. Then, to keep the aneurysm from blowing up in your face, you had to stop her heart.

Find the spot. Spread, suck, spread. Dilan probed deeper. His mind was still and sharp. He held the forceps like a pencil. The heel of his hand rested on the patient's skull. He kept his elbows pressed to his kidneys. Scrunched up like that, his arms looked undersized, like those of a T. rex. Holding yourself tight helped reduce stray movements in your fingers. He grabbed a drill with a ball-shaped bit. The bit was covered in tiny diamonds; he sheared off a piece of skull base.

"Take a little more off," Day said.

The drill whirred, high pitched. Then, like a plane dropping below the clouds, Dilan could see it all: the basilar artery, the brain stem, and next to them, the pinkish white sac of the aneurysm, gleaming and about to blow.

Arthur Day stepped in. Looking through the microscope, he examined Dilan's work. He did a small dissection to give himself a bit more room around the brain stem and then signaled to the heart team. An anesthesiologist administered a massive dose of heparin to prevent blood clots. A perfusionist manning the heart-lung machine diverted the woman's bloodstream into a box of pumps and tubes; the machine's clear tubes turned red.

Her body temperature grew colder—ninety-eight degrees, eighty . . . until it hovered at sixty. Like falling through ice on a pond— other bodily functions shut down, saving oxygen for the brain. Her systolic blood pressure dropped: sixty, fifty, forty. Her heart slowed, then stopped. Lines on the brain wave monitor went from jagged to flat; blood pressure dropped to fifteen, then zero.

Standstill.

Dilan glanced at the clock; the standstill bought them forty min- utes at most. He watched Arthur Day position the sac, which had the wrinkled look of a deflated balloon. Day picked up a Yasargil clip, invented by one of Day's teachers. The clip was the size of a mosquito. He placed it on the sac's neck.

Dilan suddenly felt uneasy. Those perforators. In the absence of any blood pressure, they had all but disappeared into the surrounding tissue. *But Art Day is a master. And what a beautiful channel he's creating with the clip.* Textbook, but not perfect enough. Dilan watched him remove the clip and try again.

Then, metal against an artery. *Did he go through one of those perforators?* No alarm, no beep or bell or profanity. The operation continued. Day finished setting the clip, then nodded to Dilan, who would close.

"Good job, everyone," Day said, as he walked out of the operating room. Dilan thought he heard a sense of defeat in his mentor's voice.

The heart team warmed her blood and restarted her heart with an electric jolt. Dilan went back to work. He sutured the meninges, the bone flap, the scalp, closing, which gave him time to think.

Failure is part of medicine, especially when you try to repair something as complex as a human brain. Failures are horrible for both patients and their doctors. But they also offer chances for redemption. If you learn from failure—if you are obsessed by it, take responsibility for it, ask yourself why it happened, always why, experience it so deeply that it feels like death—then you can forgive yourself and move forward. Then you can heal others, and in doing so heal yourself.

What would Dilan learn from this case? He wasn't sure yet. He had failed many times in the course of his training, though not always on the operating table. But he knew one thing in his heart. The woman? She would never wake up.

CHAPTER 2
———————

One year later, Dilan ducked his head through the jumbo jet's door and stepped onto the metal airport stairs. Long flight, stale airplane air, conditioned and recycled like you'd find in a hospital. He stared at the tarmac below, black as the night sky. He exhaled and then took his first breath in Tanzania. The air was sharp, a little bitter but penetrating: wood smoke, dust and plants, combustion and creation. It hit like a nicotine blast.

Since he was a brain surgeon, he knew the physiology. Molecules in the air had settled inside his nasal passages, triggering signals to the olfactory bulb, a primitive part deep in the brain, difficult to reach with your suckers and forceps. Then, neural ripples joined others, forming electrochemical waves that swept through the thalamus, the brain's switchboard, and then the two amygdalae, which form and store memories of emotional events, and finally the frontal cortex, which made sense of everything so he could say, "We're in Africa. *Aaafrica!*"

He was thirty-seven years old now, finally done with his formal neurosurgical training. He stood about six-foot-four, tall for someone in America but a giant in Sri Lanka where he was born. His skin was a rich brown, and his head was shaved, which came in handy when you explained to patients what you were about to do inside their heads. He had a prominent nose and thick, black eyebrows with sharp arches. Together, these facial angles gave him the focused appearance of an eagle. He looked particularly fierce in the operating room or outside it when lost in thought. Sometimes, he found himself telling others, "No, I'm not angry, really." He was just thinking hard about something.

When strangers learned that he was a brain surgeon, they sometimes glanced at his fingers, which were long and thin. When they shook his hand, they found it unusually warm. Conversations stopped when he walked into a room. People's eyes gravitated to him partly because of his height and shaved head but also because of his voice. It started deep in his throat, and his broad chest amplified it. He shaped words clearly with the flat vowels of South Dakota, where his family moved just before his sixth birthday. He had a habit of taking long pauses. When people asked questions, he might take a full minute to answer as he turned over the possibilities. His mother said he measured his words even when he was young because he didn't like to make mistakes. He took so long to answer that people wondered if he'd heard them in the first place. When he finally answered, he did so with conviction. This is "exactly" what should happen. This is "absolutely" the right thing to do. This procedure will be "huge."

His girlfriend of more than a year, Jenny Edwards, joined him on the tarmac. She was tall too, and athletic, with a runner's lean frame, in her fourth and final year of medical school at the University of Virginia. She had blue eyes, a tiny ring in her right nostril, and blonde hair with swirling curls. She'd listed Dilan as her fiancé on a grant application, but her left ring finger was bare. Their flight from the United States via Amsterdam had taken them through eleven time zones and at least as many squabbles.

But, a cease-fire was in effect as they joined a stream of passengers walking across the tarmac toward a long one-story building with a flat roof. Above the glass doors was a sign: Kilimanjaro International Airport. And above the sign, stars spilled out like blue-white sparks from a welder's torch.

"Look at that huge African sky!" he said.

Passports stamped, they found a taxi to Arusha.

"Open your window and smell that. Now, *that's* the smell of Africa."

His eagle look changed when he laughed and grew excited; the timbre in his voice rose; his eyebrows curved less sharply; he now looked boyish, as if about to make a dare. "We're in *Aaafrica!*"

Suddenly, it all poured into him: the scents from soil and plants, decaying and growing, the starlight, the glow from distant cook fires, the darkness. Honest things, the opposite of a modern hospital's cold fluorescent bulbs, beeping ventilators, pulse oximeters, filtered air zapped with ultraviolet rays—air never too cold or hot. In such an unchanging climate, you can grow numb to the dramas playing out inside the patients and their doctors. His jaw loosened; his long limbs relaxed. He'd waited so long for something raw and real like this, a new beginning.

They weren't yet sure how, but from Arusha they would make their way to Haydom.

The town was about 160 miles southwest on a mile-high plateau. As far as they could tell, paved roads ended just outside Arusha. The closest village was Dongobesh, about thirty miles away. It wasn't clear from the maps in his *Lonely Planet* guide whether a road connected those two towns. Maybe it was just a path. Part of him didn't want to know too much before he got there—better to just be in the moment and experience the place as things unfold. "Hey, maybe we can find a ride to Dongobesh and hike the rest of the way?" he said. He wondered if the area had lions.

He'd always wanted to go to Africa. Jenny had been leaning toward South America, but he had pressed, and she had warmed to the idea of doing her elective in Nigeria or Kenya or perhaps some country with refugees. Perfect timing. Long ago, he had promised himself that he would take time off when he finished residency, shake things up—maybe go to Sierra Leone or the Democratic Republic of the Congo. That kind of change would lay down new neural wiring over the old. But the NGOs he contacted said they didn't need brain surgeons. Are you an expert in malaria? Do you know anything about AIDS? We'd love to have you. Neurosurgeons? We're not set up to do brain surgery. The rejections had left him wondering: What happened to people with head injuries, strokes, and tumors? Refugees weren't immune to brain trauma and disease.

Then Jenny heard from a professor about Haydom Lutheran Hospital in Tanzania. They plugged the hospital's name into search engines and found bits about it here and there. Haydom wasn't on some maps, and sometimes it was spelled Haidom. Until the late 1940s, no one lived for miles around except for a man named Munya and his two wives and four sons. A group of Lutheran missionaries from Norway had built the hospital in the early 1950s. Its first doctor was named Olsen; the first four patients were construction workers who were attacked by a leopard; the hospital had four hundred beds, and 60 percent of its budget came from the Norwegian government. Bubonic plague was in the area, but more common diseases included drug-resistant malaria, tuberculosis, gastroenteritis, meningitis, parasite infections, brucellosis, and typhoid fever. A section for visiting doctors warned, "It is easy to get caught between a warm heart and a tired soul, and finding the right balance is often a personal challenge. Frustrations? You will have them!"

He'd found a phone number for the hospital and punched it in. To his surprise, the hospital's medical director picked up. His name was Oystein Olsen, grandson of the hospital's first Dr. Olsen. Over the static, Oystein said, "Of course, we'd love for you to come."

And so now they were traveling to this place, a hospital deep in the bush, hours from a paved road. He was here in Tanzania for six months—six months to figure things out.

The phone rang in their room at the Hotel Impala. Jenny picked it up: it was a British ophthalmologist also going to Haydom. Jenny looked puzzled. Neither of them knew the guy. Dilan thought, *I guess a lot of expats stay here.* The Brit said that he and a Canadian farmer had booked a small plane. It had room for two more passengers. "Meet us in the lobby tomorrow morning if you want a lift."

After Jenny hung up, Dilan asked, "Do we really want to take a plane?" He still liked the idea of hiking through the bush. But Jenny was eager to get started; she was doing this for school credit, after all.

"OK, let's do it," he said, the idea gaining purchase in his mind. Yes, flying over the bush would give him an overall feel for the place. And that's how you read CT scans and MRIs: look at the shape of a person's skull and brain structures, identify what's normal and abnormal, then zero in on things that need to be fixed.

The plane was a white single-engine Cessna with a red cross on the tail. "Flying Medical Service" was stenciled in blue on the nose. The pilot did his final checks.

Dilan folded his long legs into the copilot's seat and placed the headset over his ears. His knees pressed close to the gauges and dials. Jenny sat in the back with the eye doctor and the farmer, along with their backpacks and an emergency medical kit.

The propeller whirled, and soon they were speeding away from Arusha. Mount Kilimanjaro's snowy crown was behind them, hidden in the clouds.

As they climbed, the pilot looked ahead, no eye contact, no interest in making small talk, get it done. Which was fine. Dilan couldn't figure out how to use the headset anyway. And besides, his eyes were drawn to the colors and geology below: rusty red clays; beige mudstones; golden volcanic soils; siltstones, marls, and tuff; cashew-colored sand and darker sand like dried blood; a thousand shades of brown.

Etched here and there into these shifting shades were dark ovals. From these circles, cattle tracks and paths radiated like bent wheel spokes. His eyes traced their routes. Some shot off into the horizon. Some crisscrossed. Others split apart, and a few ended without explanation, as if a mapmaker had run out of ink. The circles turned out to be *bomas*—circular fences of thorns and bushes the Maasai used to keep wild animals out. *Awesome.* His spirits rose with every tick of the altimeter.

The land below had long fired his imagination. Looking left, he could see Tarangire National Park and the Maasai Steppe, known for their elephants, elands, and ostriches. Off to the right was the Serengeti and its wildebeest, jackals, and lions. And ahead was Lake Manyara, the lake Hemingway had written about in *The Green Hills of Africa*. Hemingway noted the lake's special "shine."

There were no green hills now. Much of the lake had dried up, leaving behind a shimmering white layer of mud and salt. But

Hemingway was right about the shine. The equatorial sun turned what was left of the shallow lake into a powerful mirror; its reflection added extra brightness to the lion-colored flanks of the Mbulu Highlands, and beyond, to the broken crater of Ngorongoro. The famous archaeologists Mary and Louis Leakey spent decades uncovering footprints, tools, and bones in nearby Oldupai Gorge. East Africa became known as the "cradle of mankind." Dilan had once thought that if he wasn't a doctor, he'd be an archaeologist. He loved digging into things, even as a child, and archaeologists had a way of getting at the sweep of it all; they hunted for answers in dirt just as surgeons did in tissues and bone. *It's all here, life, death, history; it's where everything began.*

After an hour and a half, they closed in on Mount Haydom. It was just a large hill, really, covered with oblong boulders, smooth and brown, as if someone had dropped a pile of potatoes. To the left of Mount Haydom was a dash of blond—the dried grass of the airstrip. Around it were corrugated roofs—small ones for houses and huts, and the larger red roofs of Haydom Lutheran Hospital.

"We'll circle first to chase away the goats," the pilot said. He buzzed the airstrip and pulled the plane into a tight arc. Seconds later, the plane's rubber wheels met the dry grass. Slowing now, the propeller made a sigh-like moan.

From his window, Dilan spotted people between breaks in the thornbushes. Some of the men wore blue and red blankets over their shoulders and carried long sticks. The people were tall and rail thin. They stood without moving, patient. Their faces betrayed no emotions, neither welcoming nor threatening. They stared, as if looking through the plane and its occupants to something on the horizon.

The plane stopped and the pilot cut off the engine. The door opened, and Dilan's brown Keens hit soil the color of terra cotta. As he walked away from the plane, he noticed tiny twisters of red dust curl up his pant legs. He looked at the boulders piled high on Mount Haydom, then down the length of the airstrip. He spotted dust devils far away on the plateau below. He felt the sun on his bare head, felt the openness of it all. He had a sudden urge to spread his arms wide.

A white Land Cruiser turned onto the matted grass—an ambulance from the hospital. "*Karibu,*" the driver said. Welcome.

They loaded their packs into the truck and set off down a hill, throwing up a dust wake that rose in a cloud and twisted in the slipstream. Their heads bobbed back and forth from the ruts. Small shops and kiosks lined each side of the road. Some were made of mud bricks, others with scraps of wood nailed to sticks. Shopkeepers sold pans, baskets, and pails of charcoal. A rust-colored dog loped by, its ribs as visible as jail bars. The people also seemed to be thinner than he expected. And exhausted. They lifted their legs slowly and carried herding sticks as if they were made of iron. The hospital's metal gates were at the foot of the hill, guarded by men in green military fatigues.

"A neurosurgeon," the driver said brightly. "You will be a big help in the hospital."

"Or I can chill out in the house while she works," Dilan said in jest, glancing at Jenny.

CHAPTER 3

On the globe, Africa rises like a thunderhead from the Southern Ocean, narrow at the base and 4,600 miles wide at the top. The Sahara Desert covers the uppermost part of this old land mass, as if superheated by the tropics to the south. The eastern side, meanwhile, is defined by two competing forces: tectonic plates that have been pulling apart for twenty-five million years.

The Great Rift Valley was born from this separation and friction. Like an open wound, things spilled out as the land cracked and folded, including volcanoes like Mount Kilimanjaro, and the crater Ngorongoro, and closer to Haydom, Mount Hanang. New things filled the voids: hot springs, geysers, the soda lakes of Eyasi and Natron, and Lake Tanganyika, with its lakebed 4,800 feet below the surface, the deepest in Africa.

These slow-motion forces of destruction and creation also gave plants and animals time to move to higher and lower altitudes depending on whether the globe warmed or cooled. They moved together, animal, plant, and microbe; and so on this slow-moving stage, East Africa became a place of exceptional vitality and predation.

There were leopards and hyenas, of course, but some of the most lethal predators were the smallest. Guinea worms invaded people's bodies and wiggled out of their feet. The thread-thin Loa loa migrated to the eyeball. Flatworms moved to the bladder. Tsetse flies killed livestock and gave people sleeping sickness. Swarms of mosquitoes spread malaria.

The parasites needed their human hosts, and the hosts found ways to survive, which often meant living in small family groups far apart from one another, often in highland areas above zones infested by tsetse flies and mosquitoes. People moved lightly over the land, with the animals they hunted or with small herds of cattle. Farming didn't fix them to specific plots of earth as would happen in the soil cultures of Europe and Asia. The topsoil in East Africa was often too thin anyway; the sun baked the soil hard until it fractured; high winds whisked soil and seeds into the air. When rain did come, it came in torrents; the downpours further uprooted seed sprouts and leached nutrients from the soil. In Haydom's case, the rains left behind iron oxide, creating a rusty tint.

For eons, this light human touch preserved land for animals and people alike, but it also meant that East Africa's widely dispersed groups lacked the political and military might that came with large urban centers. And this made them vulnerable to a different kind of predation: Arab slave traders first in the 1500s, followed by the Portuguese and Dutch. The Germans arrived in the late 1800s, triggering a rebellion and a vicious response. Then the British took over after World War I, the spoils of war. Independence finally came in 1961, a new layer over the old.

From Haydom, the sun rose to the left of Mount Hanang, floated for a minute as if nodding hello, and then filled the horizon with a fresh layer of orange. Three weeks after his arrival, Dilan woke up in time to see the sun's rays catch the muslin curtain above their beds and ignite it like a flame. He'd never been a morning person. Sleep was sacred. You learned that early in medical school. But he'd fallen quickly into the hospital's rhythms, so he shook away the mosquito net and swung his legs off the thin foam mattress.

Jenny was getting ready for her day on the wards, but he was in no rush. He went to the propane stove and boiled water. He poured it into a mug and added a scoop of Africafe, watching it dissolve to a deep brown. Coffee in the morning—in Africa. What could be better?

He turned around. The walls of their cottage were painted white, and the floor was polished gray cement. They had a central room with a wood-frame couch against a wall. The bathroom had a sink, a toilet, and a bathtub with no faucet. To bathe, they used a plastic bucket, filling it in the sink. Their bedroom had two single beds. He had to fold his arms and legs to fit, and the mattress was murder on his back, but overall, their cottage was more comfortable than he expected.

He joked with Jenny that he wasn't here to work, but that wasn't quite right. He desperately needed a change in his life, and one way to do that was by immersing himself in a foreign land, really dig into the place. Not treat it like a vacation. Work and live with the people. So, he would work, but on his own terms, and one of those terms was to keep the hours to a minimum so he would have time to explore or read.

He'd quickly discovered that the hospital had its own arc. Amid the birdsongs, doctors from abroad emerged from their rooms and followed paths to the dining hall. There, they sat at long communal tables and chatted in Norwegian, Dutch, and English. They sipped cups of Africafe and ate slices of Norwegian brown cheese. Then it was off to morning meetings where a Tanzanian clinical officer quietly recited names of patients who died overnight. And after that, it was off to the chapel for *Sala*, morning prayers.

He'd watched the patients arrive as the sun rose above the jacaranda trees. Patients came on foot, in wheelbarrows, on the backs of cheap Chinese motorcycles; they tumbled out of packed buses with mountains of suitcases strapped to the roofs; teams of men from deep in the Rift Valley were known to bring patients on stretchers made of animal skins.

By midday, the light was a sulfurous glare. In the dry fields around Haydom, the heat stoked those reddish-brown twisters he'd seen when he first landed. The twisters rose like wisps of smoke, whirled for a few minutes, collapsed, and reappeared nearby. In the hospital, the foreign doctors and medical students did their rounds, twisting sideways to squeeze between beds, white coats brushing against the patients' maroon blankets.

Then the descending sun cast everything in honey light, which brought out the reddish hues on Mount Haydom. From a distance, the mountain's profile looked like the shoulder hump on a bull. That's why the Datoga people called the mountain *Hay Dom*, or

Red Ox. As the air cooled, Tanzanian clinicians and nurses donned beanie caps and blankets for their walks home; patients' families lugged firewood toward the rear of the hospital to cook *ugali* over wood fires; foreign doctors returned to the dining hall to talk about the day and the safaris they hoped to do. The sky darkened and the air filled with wood smoke.

With each rotation of this cycle, Dilan felt something break free inside. It could have been simple biochemistry. When sunlight hits skin, it kick-starts production of serotonin. Low levels of serotonin in the brain affect moods, though scientists remain split over whether serotonin deficiencies trigger depression. Residency had been the definition of sun deprivation; he had spent week after week in windowless operating rooms. Now in Haydom, he felt his skin soak up the morning sun. He finished his coffee, taking one last look at the view. From the back stoop, the plateau stretched toward the horizon; acacia trees floated like smoke over the lighter browns and brightening reds of the soil. The air vibrated with the hums of bees and flies. The caffeine hit his bloodstream, sending more signals to his frontal cortex. *Yes, space, distance, the sun on my face; this is exactly what I need.*

"Hey, Dilan, what the fuck?" Arthur Day had said when Dilan told him he was taking six months off to go to Africa. Dilan had just learned some of the most challenging procedures in neurosurgery. Patients would flock to him when they learned what he could do inside their skulls. After a fellowship from Harvard, you were supposed to go to another university hospital, work like crazy for ten years, and then own the place. That was the path.

And now he was taking time off? "Why Africa?"

Another top neurosurgeon, Kim Burchiel of Oregon, had been just as blunt. "You're committing professional suicide if you go." Taking time off like this just wasn't something young neurosurgeons did. "It's going to get you away from the academic career you're trying to build. It's the first years that are important. That's when you get your grants and start building your practice."

Only John Jane, the gruff chairman of the University of Virginia's neurosurgery department, seemed to get it.

"I hear you're going to Timbuktu," he'd said with a chuckle. "You should do it. It'll make you even more interesting. But Jesus, Africa? Isn't it dangerous over there?"

CHAPTER 4

His day? First, he would head over to Radiology for the morning meeting—a good place to get an overall feel for the hospital's most pressing cases. Then, perhaps he could do a few simple spinal procedures. Brain surgery, or at least anything more complex than drilling burr holes, was out of the question. The theaters had no operating microscope. The suckers barely worked. The operating light was too dim. Patients under anesthesia were ventilated by squeezing an oxygen bag with your hands. Instruments were scattered across a storeroom that looked like a teenager's closet. He would be limited to the most basic forms of neurosurgery, which was fine with him. Just a few easy cases in the morning to keep his surgical skills sharp, and then maybe a nap or a book or a run, whatever. He would let his mind wander.

He followed a path up a hill and through a grove of jacaranda trees. Above, the limbs were mostly bare, with a few dark seedpods hanging from the branches like bats. He passed orange shipping containers stuffed with secondhand medical supplies. As he neared the wards, people nodded and smiled. Word had gotten around quickly that he was a neurosurgeon. As far as he knew, he was the first brain surgeon to visit Haydom for any length of time, perhaps ever. Prior to his arrival, Tanzania had just three practicing neurosurgeons. Three for an entire country of forty million people. And all three were in Dar es Salaam, the country's biggest city, five hundred miles away.

The United States had 3,700 neurosurgeons—not enough to keep up with the demand in either country. He didn't know it at the time, but twelve countries in sub-Saharan Africa had no neuro-surgeons at all.

He took a covered walkway to the Old Ward, which had four buildings around an open courtyard. Two large fig trees were in the center. Planted just after the hospital opened, their old roots now rose like serpents from the dirt and wound around the trunks. From the Old Ward, covered walkways led to long single-story buildings that could be easily mistaken for classrooms or military barracks. All the buildings were painted in the same two tones—beige on the upper half and red at the base to hide dust stains and mud.

Patients spilled out of open doors. Some were wrapped in blood-soaked bandages. People had fallen from bicycles or trees, and from drinking home brews of maize and honey. They had stab wounds from machetes called pangas; they had subdural hematomas after being whacked with herding staffs; they had spider and snakebites; a fourteen-year-old boy was near death from brucellosis, an infection transmitted by drinking raw milk. They had hemorrhoids, appendicitis, intestinal perforations, ruptured spleens, and hydrocephalus. Some had untreated fractures, days old, and their bones stuck out of their torn flesh. A stick-thin old man had esophageal cancer and was unable to swallow his own saliva; a woman was barely conscious after eating rat poison, probably in an attempt to commit suicide.

Dilan found himself wanting to understand the hospital's anatomy. As Arthur Day taught, go beyond the surface, ask why. Many patients had severe gastrointestinal problems, which you could trace to the lack of water treatment. About 80 percent of the water wells and holes in the area were contaminated with fecal coliform; most people simply treated water by letting it stand until the sediments settled. The wards also had a large number of epileptics. Their seizures were bad enough, but many epileptics fell into hot coals and pots of boiling sunflower oil. Burns were among the most common problems in the pediatric ward.

As far as he knew, Haydom Lutheran Hospital had never had a Tanzanian MD on its staff. Yet, the hospital seemed to have a large number of Tanzanian clinicians. Like doctors, clinical officers wore white coats and carried stethoscopes. But they had much less training. After secondary school, clinical officers typically had three years of basic clinical instruction—roughly equivalent to an American paramedic or nurse practitioner, minus a college degree. A smaller number of clinical officers went on to get two or three additional years of training and were called assistant medical officers, or AMOs.

Clinical workers and AMOs did most of the medical work in sub-Saharan Africa. Practitioners with medical degrees were rare— Tanzania had one doctor per fifty thousand people, among the worst physician-patient ratios in the world. In the United States, the ratio was about one doctor per five hundred people, and the ratios were even better in Europe. Even so, some wealthier countries had physician shortages.

As he walked past the rooms, it seemed as if every bed was occupied. Some patients slept two to a bed; some slept on floors or benches outside the rooms.

"Is the hospital always this busy?" he asked.

Yes and no, the staff said. It's always busy—the maternity ward alone delivered three to four thousand babies a year.

But the famine had made things much worse.

Across East Africa the year before, the Long Rains of March and April had mostly fallen in drips, as if the clouds had already been wrung. When storms did visit, rain fell with such force that water rolled over the soil instead of soaking into it. Seeds washed away instead of taking root. Now, a year into the drought, the red earth was dry and cracked like broken pottery. Food stores shrank, forcing farmers to buy imported grain. Grain prices doubled. "Now is hunger. People fear the sun, this sun of drought," a villager told an anthropologist.

Charities in Europe and America had taken note and pleaded for donations. When trucks full of food sacks came, word spread along the cattle tracks: "*Ufoni uaja!*" The healing has arrived!

But the food wasn't enough in many areas around Haydom. Dilan could see the evidence on the cots in front of him. Some patients had assumed the characteristics of the parched earth. They had cracked skin, cracked fingernails, and red hair—signs of malnutrition. Their thin limbs mirrored the brittle branches of the jacarandas.

Children were particularly vulnerable to diseases and parasites that prey on weakness, including tuberculosis, pneumonia, and intestinal worms. A few patients had hyena bites. Dilan had heard that the animals were moving closer to town to find food.

He felt bad for these suffering patients, but he had no urgent need to tend to them. He knew that some people found him detached, even indifferent to people's pain. In his mind, it was an occupational hazard. Neurosurgeons, despite their skills and training, often could do little for someone who had just rearranged his brain in a car wreck. His Buddhist background also affected his views of suffering. Buddhism taught that pain and suffering were inevitable, but that you could liberate yourself through meditation, mindfulness of your surroundings, compassion, and detachment from life's cravings. You don't ignore suffering. Instead, you focus on the causes and what you can and can't do to ease another person's pain. So it was in medicine: if you truly understood a disease, you could decide whether surgical intervention helped or did more harm. Often, there was nothing to be done. You let their suffering go or the enormity of it all could sweep you under.

The morning radiology meeting was about to start, but Dilan maintained his unhurried pace. He passed a line of patients along a hospital wall outside Radiology. In the waiting room, he followed a long crack in the floor that led to the office of Naftali Naman.

He'd bumped into Naman a few days before. Naman had been at his desk poring over a stack of paperwork.

"You must be the neurosurgeon. *Karibu.*"

Naman was a Tanzanian man in his fifties and had a pair of reading glasses perched on his nose. His voice was in the tenor range but had a slight rasp, as if the weight of his words were a tad too much for his vocal cords. He was the hospital's most experienced assistant medical officer. Many called him Baba Naman as a sign of respect.

"*Asante sana,*" Dilan said. Thank you. He then found himself struggling to say something else in Swahili.

"Don't worry," Naman said. "The rest of the words will follow as a matter of course. Have you seen our new CT?"

It was across the hall in a two-room suite that looked as if it had been grafted from a Western hospital. One room had a desk and two computers facing a thick pane of glass. Through that window, you could see the familiar shape of the CT scanner—the giant donut ring of X-ray tubes, and the sliding bed that went through it like a tongue depressor. Unlike other rooms in Haydom, the CT room had an air conditioner. If the air conditioner failed, Naman shut down the CT machine as well. If the CT overheated and broke, it might take months to fly in parts and technicians from Europe.

CT scanners were common enough in wealthier countries. Canada, with a smaller population than Tanzania's, had about four hundred CTs; the United States had ten thousand. But Tanzania and its forty million people had exactly three, including this one in Haydom, a used Toshiba from a hospital in Finland. The Friends of Haydom in Norway had bought it for the hospital's fiftieth anniversary the year before.

An X-ray was merely a slice of someone's bones and tissues, but a CT stacked X-rays on top of each other. Instead of a slice, you got the loaf. You could see tumors, broken blood vessels, and other land mines that might not show up on a simple X-ray. Most brain surgeons wouldn't think of operating without a CT scan, and they prefer an MRI. Tanzania had only one MRI machine, which was in Dar es Salaam. Naman talked about the CT as if it were one of his children. When Dilan had said, "This is wonderful," he meant it.

The radiology meeting was in a small room a few doors from the CT scanner. Dilan found a spot in the back. The room had seven rows of plastic chairs facing a light board. Black curtains hung over an open window. Baba Naman sat at a desk to the side and finished preparing the X-rays and CT scans for presentation. A group of European medical students walked in and took seats in the front rows. Dilan felt the muscles around his jaw tighten.

Medical students in the front rows? Sitting?

He looked around. The Tanzanian clinical officers were in the back, standing or milling about in the hallway. They had blank looks.

The Tanzanians should be in front, not the students.

Naman and a European doctor began with the day's cases, but the foreign doctors did most of the talking, often in rapid-fire bursts of accented English.

One foreign doctor rolled his eyes and sighed in exasperation.

"This is terrible, completely unacceptable." A broken bone hadn't been set properly. "This needs to be fixed now!"

Dilan thought to himself, *They're here for a few weeks, but they act like the Tanzanians are hired help.* He looked at the clinical officers again. Some stared at the floor; others stayed out in the hall.

The meeting broke with the sounds of moving chairs. A clinician he'd met earlier approached. His name was Emmanuel Mayegga.

Mayegga had a round face, almond skin, a wisp of a mustache, and a high hairline that made his forehead stand out. He'd been on call during the night when a patient with a head injury arrived. The man was barely conscious. Mayegga wasn't sure if the injury was a subdural or epidural. Either way, the man was in a bad way.

"Dr. Dilan, please, is there something you can do for this man?"

"Sure, let's go," Dilan said.

CHAPTER 5

Dilan followed Mayegga through Radiology outside to a breezeway between the hospital's buildings. To their right, patients waited next to a window to pay their bills. The surgical ward was on their left, and they entered through a heavy wooden door. Inside, patients spilled out of rooms lining both sides of a dark hallway. They found the farmer in a room with a window view of the hospital's dirt driveway. Like the other rooms, it had about twenty beds and at least as many patients. Family members stood and sat nearby. The salty and slightly metallic smell of blood mixed with the scents of soiled sheets. An open window let in dust and flies. Dilan squeezed past other patients to reach the man, who lay motionless under a maroon blanket.

He was a farmer in his early fifties. The circumstances of his injury were vague. Mayegga had heard that he'd fallen while in a stupor and bashed his head. Dilan leaned toward the man, who appeared to be unconscious. He would need to do some quick tests to calculate the farmer's Glasgow Coma Scale, a rough way of measuring the severity of a brain injury. To do that, he would need to inflict a bit of pain. He looked at Mayegga.

"Please tell him that I'm sorry."

Mayegga said a few words in Iraqw, the farmer's language and Mayegga's. Dilan clenched his fist and placed it on the farmer's sternum. Quickly, he rubbed hard, knuckles to bone. If the farmer reached for Dilan's hands to stop the pain, then his brain was in reasonably good shape. But the farmer moaned and barely moved his arms. Dilan checked his eyes. Nothing. The Glasgow Coma Scale's range is three to fifteen, with three being the worst. The farmer was a four.

"This means he's in a deep state of unconsciousness," Dilan said.

He leaned closer to the farmer's head and noticed cerebrospinal fluid dripping from one ear, another bad sign. The brain is sealed tight in the skull, and cerebrospinal fluid is part of the protective buffer between hard bone and soft brain. A leak was a life-threatening condition in itself, a vector for infections. But the drips revealed a bigger drama playing out inside the farmer's cranium. The blow to his head had breached the meninges—the brain's outer defenses—and blood and fluid had begun to pool. He could see it in his mind: the dura would be hard, stretched tight from the pressure, and purplish, like a bruise on a pale person's skin. The brain itself would have an angry red tint, like a bloodshot eyeball. Under this assault, the farmer's brain was saving energy by shutting down less vital functions: speech, movement, consciousness. His brain was probably burning glucose like crazy in a last-ditch attempt to buy more time.

"Time is brain." Dilan said this often to his surgical teams. Every minute counts when someone's brain is damaged. Fix it quickly and you might save the memory of a first bicycle ride or a family camping trip; you might save the ability to move the legs, urinate, or breathe. He could save this man. It was a simple operation. He just had to get inside his head and stop the bleeding. Except for one problem. He had no way of opening the guy's skull.

A brain weighs about three pounds. Its undulating lobes look similar to the inside of a cut-open cauliflower, but brain tissue has the consistency of brie. People sometimes describe its coloring as gray, but that's only half true. A dead brain is gray, but a live one is pinkish yellow, flush with blood. It has roughly eighty-six billion neurons, all connected in ever-changing networks. The potential combinations of these networks are the number ten followed by a million zeros. For all practical purposes, no two brains will ever be alike.

The skull is the densest bone in the body, roughly as strong as oak. The skull is thicker in some areas, such as the forehead. But near the temple in a place called the pterion, it's as thin as a cracker—no match for a smack with a stick, or a baseball, which is why baseball helmets have special flanges that extend down on the side facing the pitcher. A big artery, the middle meningeal, runs right underneath the bone. Some doctors call the pterion "God's little joke."

But any spot is vulnerable when enough force is applied to it. Even minor falls and blows could create eggshell fractures. In such cases, the skull bone bends inward from the blow but then pops back, pulled by muscles and tissue of the scalp. To the untrained eye, it might look as if nothing is amiss. But underneath the skull all sorts of mayhem can happen. If you strike your head hard enough, your brain sloshes back and forth like a sponge in a bucket. A brain has a forest of blood vessels, some as thick as cocktail straws, others finer than a strand of hair. When these blood vessels stretch and break, blood and other fluids build up inside the skull. With nowhere to go, the fluid compresses the brain, neural pathways are cut, circuits go down like a failing electrical grid.

Head injuries are as old as humanity, and so are attempts to fix them. Prehistoric healers used flints, obsidian, and other hard stones to make holes to relieve pressure, a process known as trepanation. In the 1800s doctors used chisels and mallets, often doing more harm than good. When suddenly exposed, swelling brains have a tendency to ooze out of the open skull like overbaked soufflés. Through the early 1900s, patients had a fifty-fifty chance of surviving even minor brain surgery. Because of this, the skull was sometimes called the closed box.

Harvey Cushing changed all that. Cushing was Harvard's brilliant surgeon in chief, an accomplished artist who used both hands to write on chalkboards during lectures. Instead of chisels and mallets to open a skull, Cushing carefully drilled holes with a hand trephine, a cousin of the wooden-handle corkscrew. Then he grabbed a Gigli saw, a wire with serrated edges that doctors used for amputations.

He inserted one end of the saw into the first burr hole and guided it to the second hole. He fished out the saw from the second hole and then attached T-shaped handles to both ends. He moved the saw back and forth, as if flossing a tooth. When the wires met, he'd cut a line in the skull. Doing this in a circle, he could pop off a patch of skull like the top of a jack-o'-lantern.

The procedure was called a craniotomy, and with this technique, Cushing was able to expose the brain without turning it into a bloody pulp—he opened the closed box.

Gigli saws were still available, low tech, and cheap—twenty bucks in the United States. Some neurosurgeons used them even when they had electric or pneumatic saws at their disposal; they liked the feel of the wires and the back-and-forth rhythm. Dilan had an unproven theory: if given a choice, most neurosurgeons would choose manual transmissions over automatics.

Because Gigli saws were used for amputations, Dilan had thought the hospital might have one socked away in a storeroom and had gone looking for one as soon as he arrived. He opened cabinets and drawers, rifled through closets and boxes stuffed with secondhand supplies. He found suction tubes, clamps, retractors, dissectors, scalpels, and a Hudson Brace, a hand drill that looked like an eggbeater, all of which could be used in neurosurgery. But no Gigli saw.

Then, while searching a storage room, he discovered an old wooden case. The wood was honey-colored with long, dark grains, burnished by use and time, probably brought by a European doctor decades ago. The case had two brass hinges and a brass clasp. He opened it, and there it was: a Gigli saw, coiled in a circle and held in place by four wood blocks.

It looked like a museum exhibit, as if the nineteenth-century doctor Leonardo Gigli had made it himself. Dilan picked it up. It was rusty and broken into several pieces. *How cool is this to find something so old?* He studied it more closely.

You could use it if it was rusty—just clean and sterilize it—but not if it was broken or so weakened by rust that it might break inside a patient's skull. This was both rusty and broken. He had put the saw away and closed the box. *Awesome.* But no use at all. Beyond repair.

CHAPTER 6

Dilan couldn't help the farmer, so he decided to go for a run—keep the work-life balance in check. Back at the cottage, he slipped into his shorts and put on his brown Nikes. He followed the long driveway to the gates. To the right, a small building sold gospel music and Bibles. Ahead, a steady stream of people moved through the swinging gates. In any given hour, six hundred might pass through: tall men with spines as straight as their staffs; children in green-and-maroon school uniforms; nursing students in pink uniforms and black shoes. People wore sandals made from old tire treads, yellow flip-flops, rubber wading boots, formal black-leather shoes. Dilan nodded to the gate guards, and then he was outside.

Across the road was a stall with a sign that said Junction Shop. Next to it was a cobbler sitting on a plank beside a sign that said Dr. Shoes. An uneven line of shops and huts ran up the hill, with empty spots here and there, like a mouthful of bad teeth. The road had been baked so hard that its surface had split into jagged fissures. He noticed again the slow pace of people around him and the exhausted lopes of the dogs. Everything and everyone seemed to be waiting for the rain to return, except perhaps the children.

On the way up the hill, kids emerged from the doors of huts and shop stalls. They ran a few steps toward him with grins. They shouted, "*Mzungu! Mzungu!*" It was Swahili for "white person" or "foreigner." Its etymology was thought to be rooted in the phrase "wander or spin in circles," which is what European explorers and traders appeared to do when they first came to this land. But Tanzanian children shouted it as if they'd seen a celebrity. Older people occasionally used it less charitably, depending on the context and particular *mzungu*. But, overall, it didn't seem to carry the same baggage as other racial labels.

Just the same, he didn't like labels. On himself and others. Yes, his skin was brown, but he sometimes thought of himself as white, given his upbringing in the States. Yet he also was deeply attached to his native Sri Lanka. White? Asian? In his mind, what did it matter? People often comfort themselves by dividing people into groups that fit their own worldviews. He had no interest in promoting such comfort. Tanzanians and Europeans at the hospital often asked whether he was from Ethiopia or Somalia.

"No."

"India?"

"Good guess," he would say, and then change the subject.

He reached the top of the hill and turned right, passing between the thornbushes that guarded the airstrip. High, flat, and open, the airstrip felt like a stage. The midday sun was a powerful spotlight. He felt as if his eyes had gained extra contrast.

That farmer? He would die soon. *Nothing I can do. Let it go.*

A stiff wind blew. He felt the dust on his pores. What a relief it was to have no responsibilities for a change. He took off down the airstrip, light steps, then faster.

Midway, something caught his eye. A bush. It was shaking in a violent way. Couldn't be the wind. Nothing else was around. Hyenas? You could see their chalky white turds around the airstrip.

Then he saw two arms coming out of the bush, moving back and forth like pistons.

Closer, and he saw the full figure of a man cutting a tree limb with a wire saw.

The man was tall and had a *shuka* blanket draped over his shoulder.

"*Jambo*," Dilan said, still wishing he knew more Swahili. He used hand signals and a few other Swahili words to ask where the man had bought the saw.

"Mbulu," the man said.

It might take a day or two to figure out how to get there and back.

Dilan asked if he could look at the saw.

The man handed it to him. It was about two-and-half-feet long with three thin strands twisted around each other to create a jagged cutting edge.

"Can I buy this?"

The man looked puzzled.

More hand movements followed as Dilan offered the man twenty thousand shillings, about fourteen dollars, close to what he would pay for a saw online in the States, about two weeks of income for the average person around Haydom.

The man handed over his saw, his face a mix of bemusement and triumph.

Dilan coiled it and turned back toward the hospital. *Time is brain.*

Through the late 1800s, hospitals in North America and Europe were chaotic places, crowded with patients in various states of agony and infection. During surgeries, apprentice surgeons climbed on nearby beds to watch the carnage. With no good pain medication, operations resembled wrestling matches. Orderlies pinned patients to tables while doctors sliced open body cavities or amputated limbs. Speed was paramount.

Robert Liston was Britain's best surgeon in the mid-1800s and was known to do amputations in under a minute. "Time me, gentlemen; time me," he said before operations. Once when amputating a patient's leg, he accidentally sliced off an assistant's finger, and while switching instruments, slashed a spectator. The patient and assistant later died from infections, and the spectator was said to have died of shock; it was the only operation known to have a 300 percent mortality rate.

If patients survived their surgeries, they still had to contend with infections, possibly from a previously used bandage or from a doctor who wore the same bloodstained coat day after day. As late as 1875, Bellevue Hospital in New York had a sign above operating tables with six-inch letters written in black: PREPARE TO MEET YOUR GOD.

As fascination about surgery grew, hospitals built amphitheaters, some big enough to hold 450 people. Operations became high-stakes entertainment, and surgeons were the stars. Writing about an operation at Bellevue in the 1870s, a New York physician described how a surgeon's knife "glittering for a moment above the head of the operator was plunged through the limb, and with one artistic sweep, made the flaps and completed the circular amputation. The fall of the amputated part was greeted with tumultuous applause by the excited students. The operator acknowledged the compliment with a formal bow."

Surgical amphitheaters began to disappear in the late 1800s and early 1900s as scientists learned more about bacteria and infections. Yet many hospitals in Europe and Africa still used the term *operating theater* instead of the more mundane *operating room*. And surgeons were still stars. Surgeons often talked about the need to be bold; when they saw a threat, such as an aneurysm or a tumor, they had to act. Laziness or indecision could kill. Donald Effler, one of the first doctors to do open-heart surgery, said, a great surgeon "must have a driving ego, a hunger beyond money. He must have a passion for perfectionism. He is like the actor who wants his name in lights." At Harvard, Arthur Day sometimes opened a skull and announced, "This is the stage!" Likewise, Dilan preferred the term *theater*. When it came to brain surgery, even the smallest slip could leave a patient paralyzed or dead. And what was more dramatic than putting your fingers into someone's mind?

The farmer was on a table in Theater One. Dilan had sorted through a bin of green scrubs, trying to find an extra large. The pants he found rode high on his ankles. His scrub top felt tight around his armpits. He scrubbed his hands in one of the three sinks outside the theater. Masks dangled from a shelf to the right. He shook the water droplets off his hands and walked through a double door.

The theater's floor was concrete—gray and polished. The equipment was old, but the room was remarkably clean. The walls were white, and the ceiling had two bare fluorescent tubes. Four chains dangled from the ceiling with wire cages for glass IV bottles. Two screen windows let in the breeze. A black plastic clock tilted on the wall, ticking.

Since the theater's lights were so dim, Dilan strapped his camper's headlamp around his forehead. He worked with a nurse to put a tray together. He gave instruments simple names: "big biter" for the Leksell and Adson rongeurs and "nibbler" for the smaller Lempert rongeurs. He had the tree saw sterilized in an autoclave across the hall. The wire lay coiled next to the other instruments like a dark snake.

Victor, a Tanzanian anesthesiologist with a thin mustache and sleepy eyes, manned an oxygen bag. He squeezed it gently, ventilating the farmer's lungs. Standing behind Dilan was Emmanuel Mayegga, there to observe. A nurse stood by with an orange flyswatter.

"Is the suction working?" Dilan asked the nurse.

The nurse nodded yes, but not in a confident way. No problem. If the suckers failed, he'd sop it all up with gauze.

He rolled a stiff green towel into a tube and shaped it into a loop. He placed the loop under the farmer's head to make a cradle. He didn't want the man's head to move when he drilled.

A nurse shaved the farmer's head and smeared grain alcohol on the incision site. Normally, Dilan used a black pen to outline where he would make his first cuts. But he didn't have a pen so he used a needle. He scratched a reverse question mark in the farmer's scalp. The needle tip made a thin white line. He took a No. 10 scalpel and made a quick inch-long cut, following the line's curve. Then another. He retracted the skin and scraped away a layer of muscle, revealing bone.

Now the Hudson drill. His left hand held the handle, his right found the crank. He moved the bit over the bone, pressed, and cranked; the gears squeaked; white bone dust piled up around the hole. He made another hole an inch away, then inserted a thin metal strip called a brain protector between them. The strip would shield the brain from the tree saw's edges; he'd found it in the garage next to other ambulance parts. *Good*, he thought. *The mechanics did a nice job cutting it to size.*

Leaving the brain protector in place, he inserted the wire saw at an angle, making sure it went between the brain protector and the skull. When the end appeared by the second hole, he pulled it through. Then, Harvey Cushing style, he lifted both ends and moved the wire back and forth, cutting the bone.

Cool, it's working.

He drilled more holes, sawed back and forth, until he could open the farmer's hood.

Just in time. The brain was badly swollen. It had that angry red and purple coloring and was full of blood and cerebrospinal fluid.

Dilan found the damage and used an electric cauterizing tool to stop the bleeding. The tool zapped and sizzled and sent up wisps of smoke. The smoke smelled like burned hair. He flushed the wound with saline. He watched the farmer's bruised brain pulse. With Emmanuel Mayegga still watching, he reversed what he'd done, closed the box.

"Nothing to it," he said, and walked out the door.

Victor, the anesthesiologist, continued to squeeze and release the ventilating bag. He'd seen hundreds of patients with head injuries die because no one could help them. As he watched Dilan leave, he said under his mask, but loud enough for Mayegga to hear, "We have a neurosurgeon."

CHAPTER 7

Dilan ditched his green scrubs in the changing room and followed the breezeway back to the hospital's entrance. "Wow," he kept telling himself. "I just used a tree saw to open someone's skull."

Adrenaline coursed like electricity through his bloodstream, that familiar jolt from doing something new, of solving a problem that others hadn't. He felt his feet scrape the dirt, felt the clean, dry air in his lungs. After a surgery like this, his senses came alive. Sometimes it even felt like joy.

With a CT scanner and a wire saw, he had opened the closed box. That meant he could repair subdural hematomas, drain abscesses, remove meningiomas and other tumors. Suddenly he had a caseload of patients who otherwise would have died. More patients than one neurosurgeon could ever handle.

On the way back to the cottage he passed the eye clinic and then the steps to the hospital library. *A decent little library*, he thought. It had rare articles about the area's history and old textbooks on tropical diseases. A fun place to spend a few hours and pull out books at random. But it also reminded him of the medical students, the ones who sat in the front during radiology meetings. *What the fuck?* The foreign students did the same thing during the morning report, which was usually held in the library. They walked in as if they owned the place and took seats around the tables in the center of the room. The Tanzanians mostly stood behind them.

He found himself thinking more about the morning report. It was a waste of time—just a recitation of those who died and who had been admitted. In teaching hospitals across North America, morning report was a jolt of caffeine. Residents and students presented cases. Senior doctors fired questions at you like bullets. You returned fire just as quickly with crisp answers. Hesitation was a sign of weakness. These interrogations were called pimping. And they were done within a strict hierarchy: senior doctors asked questions first to the least experienced students and residents in the room, and if they didn't know the answers, they moved up the food chain to junior residents and sometimes the chief. Pimping was an active way of learning and teaching, a way to sharpen the blade. But there was nothing sharp about the morning report here. No transfer of knowledge. And in a library, of all places. A subroutine from residency played in his mind: every conversation about a patient is an opportunity to learn. Every chance to learn is a chance to save a life.

Near the jacaranda trees, Dilan spotted Oystein Olsen, the medical director. Oystein greeted him with a handshake and a look that suggested he had something on his mind.

Oystein was in his early forties with straight blond hair parted neatly on the side. His eyes were blue, and he had blond eyebrows that seemed to generate their own light. He was Haydom's third Dr. Olsen. His grandfather, Olaf Olsen, had been the first, arriving in 1954 with his wife, Borghild, as the Old Ward went up. Oystein's father, Ole Halgrim Evjen Olsen, was the second Dr. Olsen and arrived with his wife, Mama Kari, in December 1961, the day after the country gained its independence. The second Dr. Olsen had died of cancer just a few months before Dilan's arrival, but Mama Kari still lived in their house on the hill. She toured the grounds with her metal walker and invited visitors for cakes and tea.

Oystein was clearly a different missionary than his father and grandfather—more cerebral, less hands-on. He often talked about the importance of trust in medicine and what he thought was an overemphasis on disease prevention. A huge infrastructure had been created to combat malaria, AIDS, and tuberculosis—important work. But that didn't help a mother who lost her child because no obstetrician was there to do a C-section, nor did it help the boy who became an invalid after a motorcycle accident because a trauma doctor wasn't available to set his bones. Families who lost loved ones because of this dearth of doctors also lost trust in the hospital. Without trust, desperate patients might seek out traditional healers, or seek no help at all. A trustworthy hospital did as much as it could on all fronts, not just hand out mosquito nets, vaccines, and antiretrovirals.

Which is why he'd been so pleased at first that Dilan was visiting Haydom. If you demonstrated to your patients that you could do brain surgery, well, that would send a message about the hospital's competence in more mundane areas: delivering babies, fixing bowel obstructions, treating pneumonia. It would build trust.

But he had something other than brain surgery on his mind when he greeted Dilan that afternoon.

"We want you to be a more active part of the hospital," Oystein said, getting to the point. "We want you to take call." He didn't have to spell out what he really meant: Dilan wasn't working hard enough.

Dilan laughed. Taking call meant doing everything from treating snakebites to diagnosing malaria.

"I haven't delivered a baby since medical school. You really need to talk to Jenny. She's the one who's here to work."

Oystein pressed. "It would be really helpful. We want our visiting doctors to share their knowledge. The hospital is very short-staffed."

"Yeah, I'm sorry. There's no way I'm taking call."

They left it that way. You can't order a volunteer to work.

Dilan followed the hill down to his cottage. He felt a chill in the air. Haydom had thin topsoil. With the sun gone, the red earth quickly gave up its heat.

He wouldn't hold it against Oystein for trying to squeeze more work out of him. The hospital could use a dozen more doctors.

But why not do more with the Tanzanian clinical officers?

The hospital seemed to have plenty on its staff.

No, he wasn't here to do someone else's job.

No one knew he was in Africa to save himself. No, for them to truly understand, they would need to experience medical school and residency themselves, take the insane tunnel that Jenny was about to enter, the one that nearly destroyed him.

CHAPTER 8

If he looked back, really far back, the entrance to that tunnel wasn't residency. It was Sri Lanka, which was still called Ceylon when he was born.

His father, Somisara, was a gregarious man with a small tuft of black hair. He taught middle and high school in the mountain city of Kandy. When teaching, he often opened his eyes wide when making points, as if shocked, and then narrowed them as if savoring something delicious. Somisara loved teaching but also dreamed of lands beyond Sri Lanka. Then, in 1956, he won a three-month Fulbright grant to study in the United States. Because he was interested in agriculture, he chose South Dakota State in America's farming heartland. He'd quickly made friends there who urged him to immigrate. But he had his parents to tend to back home, so he returned to Sri Lanka, part of him wondering if he should have stayed in the United States.

Back in Kandy, Somisara was in a bookstore one day when he spotted a beautiful young woman in a blue sari. Her name was Chitra. She had butterscotch skin and was about five-foot-six, unusually tall in Sri Lanka; her friends called her Skyscraper. She, too, was a teacher—physics and math at a nearby high school.

They eventually married and settled in a small house above Kandy Lake. They had a daughter, Vayomi, which means "I am air," and a second they called Hemali, "golden rays of the sun." Dilan was born in 1969, a rare name that means "two lands."

As a child, he had fine black hair, his father's clear eyes, and big round ears that stuck out like two open clamshells. He'd shown an early ability to focus on a goal, an unusual stubbornness. He cried and refused to sleep unless he had his favorite pillow, the one made from cotton puffs from his grandfather's garden. For a long time, he wore only one shirt, a yellow T-shirt with a line of kangaroos hopping after each other. When he was four, he found a small crack near the front door. He took his pointer finger and pressed into it. Dust came out, and he pressed harder. He did this for days. As more dust came out, he realized he was making the crack much bigger, which was wonderful. If you kept at it, you could change something as big and permanent as a wall. It was his first surgery.

Not long after that, he told his parents, "I'm going to be a doctor, just like my uncle. And I'm going to be tall, even taller."

He said this smiling with pride, as if he had drawn something beautiful.

Dilan wouldn't know until much later, but his announcement had a profound effect on his parents. Both had grown restless. His father had quit teaching for a time to run a cereal factory. His mother feared that her children weren't getting proper educations. The government put children into career tracks, and Dilan's oldest sister ended up in a math and science track even though she was better suited to art and literature. Bribes could change their children's paths, but his father grew furious at the thought of paying someone off. Yet, without bribes, Dilan would likely never become a doctor in Sri Lanka. His parents decided they would move to America.

But he and his sisters loved Kandy and all its colors and smells. Buddhist monks in orange and yellow robes walked with unhurried deliberation through the streets. In the back of the house, monkeys peeled off roof tiles and played with their drying clothes. Mangos and passion-fruit vines grew by their house. During the festival to honor the Sacred Tooth, streets were lined with torches that burned coconut husks; dancing boys tossed batons of fire; and hundreds of elephants marched through, their backs and enormous ears adorned with colorful cloth and sparkling with tiny electric lights.

And now, they were being told they had to leave this storied place.

But in America, everything is possible, his father said. A doctor? You'll be in the country that just sent a man to the moon. You could become anything you wanted there: an astronaut, a doctor. All you had to do was work hard and focus on your goal.

They kept their departure secret. Brain drain was a problem, and the government was trying to prevent educated people from leaving. So in late December 1974, they quietly sold and gave away most of their belongings to pay for tickets and packed the rest in a few suitcases. They said good-bye to the rest of their family and the shimmering emerald hills of Kandy.

They would fly to Russia, then Canada, and finally the United States. His father had just twenty dollars stuffed in his sock. Dilan was a few days from turning six. He left his kangaroo shirt behind but held his favorite pillow tight, a boy now of two lands.

Of course, lots of kids say they will be doctors when they grow up. It sounded important. It set you apart from other children. As a child, he thought to himself, *If I become a doctor, then everyone will know I'm a good person.* Smiles from adults reinforced this goal. They would say, "A doctor! Wonderful!" In Sri Lankan culture, being a doctor was particularly prized. The third-century king Buddhadasa was thought to have done brain surgeries, and said, "If you can't be king, be a healer."

But what turns a dream into resolve? In Dilan's mind, part of the answer lay in his parents' decision to move to America. They left family and friends behind for him and his sisters. He would find some way to honor their sacrifice.

They arrived in Brookings, South Dakota, after seeing their first snow in Russia and their first escalators.

They were on foreign soil but almost immediately among friends. During his father's Fulbright visit in 1956, he'd met a Greek man named Gus Kakonis. Kakonis had owned a café then and invited Somisara and other Fulbright scholars to use the kitchen to cook their native cuisines.

Now, eighteen years later, Kakonis was driving them across the prairie to Brookings, where he owned the Pizza King. Dilan's parents would manage the restaurant. Kakonis also had a one-bedroom apartment directly above. That's where they would live.

They found the closets in their new apartment stuffed with warm clothes donated by Kakonis and his friends. The kitchen was stocked with dishes and pans. A reporter for the daily paper stopped by to write about his father's "love affair" with Brookings, and how it had ended happily with his return. "I was foolish to go back" to Ceylon in 1956, he told the reporter, then paused, and as he did with his children, turned his comment into a question: "Was I foolish to go back?"

Soon, the scents of Chitra's curries blended with the restaurant's tomato sauce and dough. Dilan and his sisters watched *Little House on the Prairie* in their little apartment on the prairie. His parents slept in the bedroom, and he and his sisters slept together in the dining room behind a divider. He was growing so fast by then that his arms and legs ached. Some nights he couldn't sleep because of the pain, even with his favorite pillow.

But like that pillow, he held firmly to his plan to be a doctor. The more he dreamed about it, the more convinced he became of his goal's merits. If he became a doctor, he would be important, one worthy of respect, maybe even a wealthy man. He would be someone who made others feel better, a good person.

His future status as a doctor became expected, part of the family's muscle memory. One day not long after they moved, he and his father went to the local school's oval track. Dilan was tall and fast and could beat many of his playmates in races.

"I think you will be a good athlete," his father said. "If you're fast enough, you can get a scholarship."

"I want to be a doctor. I won't have much time for sports," Dilan replied.

"That means you will have to do very well in science. And you will have to cultivate deep concentration, and that means keeping your mind on a single thought."

"That's hard, but I'll try. Which colleges are best?"

Harvard and Yale were tops, he said. Harvard was like Trinity in Sri Lanka, and Yale was like Royal, Trinity's archrival.

His father had gone to Trinity.

"I want to go to Harvard, not Yale. I want to be a doctor at Harvard." And then his father sent him off to run laps.

·   ·   ·

But resolve gets you only so far. In Brookings, he also learned that fear and anger could change your trajectory. With the exception of a few Native Americans, nearly everyone in Brookings was white, mostly of German and Norwegian stock. He'd shortened his name from Dilantha to Dilan, pronounced "deh-lahn," though people invariably called him Dylan, like the musician. When people asked Dilan and his sisters where they were from, they said Ceylon and usually got blank faces in return. They said it was near India. More blank looks.

His oldest sister, Vayomi, was tall and striking and quickly fit in at high school. But the middle sister, Hemali, had left many friends behind in Sri Lanka, and now here she was in a foreign country, stuck in middle school with no friends at all. Kids tripped her in the hallways, stuck gum in her hair, and called her "nigger toad." She grew sullen and quiet and retreated into books and television. Dilan heard the same taunts at his school.

"Nigger, nigger," said James, a blond boy, in a singsong way.

"Nigger, nigger," a huge Native American boy chimed in.

The taunts continued for months. He told his teachers, but the boys were careful to call him names when adults weren't around. His parents met with teachers. Nothing changed.

One afternoon, he climbed onto the apartment's roof. He went there to think sometimes. Vayomi saw that something was bothering him and joined him. She listened to him talk about the bullies and how he couldn't stop them. His father overheard their conversation and asked them to come down.

"Violence is always wrong," he said. "But in some cases, if you don't speak the same language as the other person, you're not going to get your message across."

During the summer, he taught Dilan how to throw and block punches and to stay away from the groin; gentlemen didn't hit in that area. When school started that fall, Dilan hoped the boys would stop. But they came at him again.

"Nigger, nigger."

One day as recess ended, he hid around the corner of the school building and waited. Soon, a straggler passed by—James, the short, stocky kid with blond hair and a sharp nose.

Dilan popped out from the corner, grabbed him by the jacket, and pulled him out of sight of the teachers. He pushed James up against the wall.

"If you call me nigger again, I'm going to hit you until you can't get up again. Do you understand?" All James could do was nod and say, "Yes, I understand."

The next day Dilan waited behind the corner again. Another boy passed, and he grabbed him. This boy resisted, and Dilan punched him in the mouth. The boy fell to the ground.

"If you call me nigger again, I'm going to hit you until you can't get up again. Do you understand?"

Dilan picked off three other boys in the same fashion until only one remained, the Native American boy. But he was so big that he could easily make Dilan's face look like a Pizza King pie. He'd have to do something different.

He saw a chance when he spotted him during gym class, alone on a bench watching the other kids play basketball.

"You're the same color as I am, and you're calling me nigger. If you keep calling me nigger, then I'm going to call you nigger, and then there will be two of us. Do you want that?"

The kid said nothing, just glared. Dilan feared they would all gang up on him.

But within a day everything changed. The bullies suddenly became his friends, even the ones he'd punched, even the huge Native American boy. They invited him to their homes. Instead of being afraid and frustrated, he had buddies. The change was so sudden that it was magical. It hardwired something into his brain that years later would help him become a doctor: use your resolve to set a goal, and then take action. Be methodical about reaching it, be precise, but don't just stand there. Take action, and you can turn fear and anger into success. Do it, and anything is possible.

Anything is possible here. I could even become an astronaut. But I'm going to be a doctor. As he grew older, this resolve gained more gravity. He wouldn't be just any doctor. He'd be *the best doctor*, one who treated others as if they were *his* family.

Other teens plastered walls with posters of rock groups and sports icons, but Dilan taped a black-and-white photo of a surgeon on his door. The surgeon had gray hair and a chiseled face. A mask dangled below his chin. His eyes were on fire with concentration and triumph. *Who wouldn't be pumped after saving someone's life?* Later, when school counselors asked about his backup plans if he didn't get into medical school, he looked at them as if they'd spoken Dutch.

He enrolled at the University of Washington, majored in psychology, then was accepted to its medical school. He came across a book called *To Be a Surgeon* by a heart surgeon named Richard Furman. Furman described how he began his quest in high school by scribbling on a sheet of paper "Set your goals high," and once you identify a major goal, "Set It, and Never Change It."

Yes, Dilan thought, here's someone who believes in goals as much as I do.

Yes, a goal was a start. But a goal without action was useless. It was worse than useless; it was a phantom, real but in your mind, haunting you about your failures. The only way to get rid of that ghost was to do something, get it done, like he'd done with those bullies.

He would master medical school the same way he'd taken care of the bullies: break tasks into parts, practice them until they became second nature, then do more than his superiors ever expected. During rotations, a typical medical student might examine four patients and present their vitals during the morning meeting. He went in at 3 a.m., examined forty-five patients, memorized their vitals using index cards, changed into a fresh white jacket, always pressed, then presented the patients' information, all from memory, no index cards, hands behind his back. Get it done.

A dream was one thing, but spending a decade and a half chasing it was another. That's how long it took to become a brain surgeon in the United States: five years of medical school, research, and an internship, then six to eight years of residency, plus another year or two doing a fellowship. Talk about a long tunnel.

Doubts came in medical school. *Sure, if I try hard enough, I'll become a surgeon. But what will it do to me?*

He saw clues in the operating rooms—how residents and attending doctors bragged about their affairs and sexual escapades. At his own hospital at the University of Washington, a neurosurgeon took students on car rides and purposely blew through red lights. The message was clear: neurosurgeons worked on people's brains; waiting at red lights was for mortals. When Dilan interviewed for residency programs, he heard people at Duke speak with pride about the department's 100 percent divorce rate. At Baylor, he heard about an imaginary red line around the ICU. The story went that residents doing their ICU rotation weren't allowed to step over that line for weeks. When one resident crossed the line to meet his wife in the parking lot, he was fired the next day. Dilan wasn't sure whether these stories were true. But the smirks as they talked about their failed relationships told him plenty about the mind-set.

One day in medical school he shadowed a chief resident, a guy in his final year of neurosurgical training, top of the residency food chain. They were in the hallway of Seattle's Harborview Hospital. An ambulance had just delivered a seventeen-year-old girl to the ER. A bad car wreck. Members of her family were up ahead, waiting for word.

Dilan stood to the side and watched the chief walk toward them, stop, and in a monotone, say, "She has a severe brain injury. The chances of her living are almost none." He said a few more words in the same flat voice, then turned ninety degrees and walked down another hallway.

Dilan watched the family wither. The chief hadn't introduced himself, asked them their names, or taken them to a side room to break the worst news they might ever hear. And then he'd just turned his back on them and left. They would forever remember that moment, the day one of the most important people in their lives had died and how indifferent the doctor had been to their loss. Scientists called these indelible moments "flashbulb memories." *If I become a neurosurgeon, will I become an asshole like him?*

He had a choice, after all. He didn't have to go into neurosurgery.

One sunny afternoon, he found his father in the backyard.

"I'm thinking about doing family medicine or neurosurgery," he said. "I like working with patients and their families, and family doctors do only three years of residency. If I did family medicine, I'd have a life, and I'd still be helping people. But if I do neurosurgery, that could take nine years. I'd have no life."

His father pondered his son's predicament for a few long moments.

"Then you should be a family doctor. You should have a life."

CHAPTER 9

But Dilan had fallen in love with the brain, hard. Some days, he snatched one from a lab, put it in a glass jar, and took it back to his apartment. He pulled it out at random times and held it up to the light. He studied the curves of the occipital lobe in the back, the pineal gland, shaped like a tiny pinecone. "It's all so beautiful," he'd say, and then to his roommate's disgust, he'd put the brain back in the fridge with the other leftovers.

Then one day a senior resident invited him to observe a tumorectomy. Dilan watched the resident open the patient's skull, and there it was, a live brain. Instead of the hard gray brain in his jar, this one was pink and gleaming, pulsating in tandem with the patient's heart.

"Do you want to touch it?"

"Absolutely." Hesitation was a sign of weakness.

"OK, squirt some water on your gloves. You don't want your finger to stick."

Dilan moistened the fingertip of his surgical glove. He moved his pointer finger closer, feeling as if he were about to set off the hospital's fire alarm. Then his fingertip touched the patient's brain. He pushed harder. It was the consistency of tofu, and he could feel it vibrate. Time seemed to slow. He touched it for maybe ten seconds, but as he left the OR, he felt as if he'd landed on another shore. It was so sensual, but not in a sexual way. You were touching a person's past and dreams, everything a person is and would be. He hadn't expected the experience to be so intimate; touching another person's brain was more profound than making love.

.   .   .

But could he actually operate on something so easily damaged, so complex? One day in medical school, a neurosurgeon named Kai Johansen asked if he wanted to observe a carotid artery operation.

"Absolutely."

The carotid artery curved across the fold of the man's neck like a road up a mountain. Johansen's job was to cut it apart, clean out the blockages, and put it back together.

"Your turn," he told Dilan.

"I'm sorry, what?"

"Cut the artery."

"I can't do that. I'm just a medical student."

"Anything you fuck up, I can fix."

He picked up a scalpel from the tray. He looked at the artery, illuminated by a spotlight. He watched his hand move toward the neck and cut the artery. It bled just like the textbook said it would. He worked on the artery for an hour, though it seemed like just a few minutes. He heard Johansen's gruff voice: "Close it up."

When he was done, he'd crossed another divide. Before, he believed that he could do brain surgery.

Now he *knew* he could do it.

Like love, the brain could also break your heart. Just before graduation, he landed a neurosurgery rotation at a hospital in New York. A chief resident asked if he wanted to do a biopsy.

"Absolutely."

It was a simple procedure: drill into the skull and pluck out a piece of tissue. The woman's scalp was cut back. He picked up the hand drill. It had a crank on one side. Its bit was designed to catch just as it went through the bone. He placed the bit against her skull and turned the handle. He pressed harder, turned the crank faster. It broke through but didn't catch. He felt the bit drive into the woman's brain.

"Let me see," the attending said, moving Dilan aside.

Waves of nausea shot across his stomach and up through his chest, sucking air from his lungs.

"Let's take the biopsy," the attending said. He removed the specimen and closed, and then a CT scan was taken. The doctors and Dilan filed into a room for a look. And there it was on the computer screen, his mistake: a shaft-like void in the woman's brain.

He was with her when she woke up. She had trouble moving her arm. "I'm sorry you're weak after this," he said, without going any further. The attending physician had decided against a full explanation. Dilan visited her every two hours, stayed with her late into the night and early the next day. The biopsy results came back: malignant. At best, she had a few months to live. And he had made this time that much harder.

The chief resident took him aside. "This happens once or twice a year. Don't beat yourself up about it."

"Thanks," he said, but he felt as if someone had scraped off his stomach lining. This was more than guilt; it was a dagger.

He replayed what happened. He was going too fast. He was pressing too hard. He didn't know what it felt like to stop once the drill was about to break through. He was trying to impress everyone. *Am I a horrible person? Should I be a neurosurgeon? How can I live with this?*

Forgive and Remember was the title of another book that changed his life. A sociologist named Charles Bosk had spent years at a hospital in San Francisco trying to understand what made surgeons tick. In one study, Bosk interviewed a group of neurosurgical residents who had been fired or left for other reasons and then compared their responses to those who finished their residencies. He'd noticed a pattern. Those who had dropped out or been fired often blamed other people for operating room mistakes or blamed fate or the patients themselves; they hedged and gave imprecise answers to direct questions.

Successful residents, on the other hand, were quick to admit what they had done wrong, often going into great detail about exactly how they had screwed up. Bosk concluded that dexterity wasn't a deciding factor in what made successful neurosurgeons; rather it was an obsession with failure. That's how great surgeons lived with themselves. They forgave but remembered.

Dilan's father was probably right. If he wanted to have a life, he should graduate from medical school and do his residency in family medicine.

And yet, the brain! Such a challenge. So delicate and personal. Life or love?

He chose love.

CHAPTER 10

It didn't always take so long to become a surgeon. Until the mid-1800s, surgeons learned their skills by apprenticing a year or two or by attending the equivalent of a trade school. At some schools, applicants simply had to know how to read and write. All this changed in large part because of William Stewart Halsted.

Dilan and most every other doctor who went through residency knew about Halsted and could trace their suffering and their success to him.

Halsted was a fastidious dresser who kept his fine, light hair parted in the middle and well oiled. In the 1870s he was one of New York's best young surgeons, a doctor who "worked with superhuman energy and endurance," according to one biographer. And, he was a quick thinker. When his pregnant sister began to hemorrhage, he grabbed a syringe, plunged the needle into his own arm, withdrew blood, then inserted the needle into hers—the first successful blood transfusion in the United States.

Then, Halsted began experimenting with cocaine. Thinking correctly that it would make a good local anesthetic, he and several colleagues tested it on each other. Within a few weeks all were addicted. Several later died from overdoses. Over time, Halsted's life unraveled. In 1885 he was scheduled to do a surgery at Bellevue on a construction worker who had broken his legs. Halsted entered the operating room, touched the patient's leg, and then ran out the door. It was the start of a seven-month stupor. He eventually sought refuge in a rehabilitation facility in Rhode Island, which treated his withdrawal symptoms with morphine. Halsted soon fell under morphine's spell and would spend the rest of his life balancing his highs and lows with both drugs.

Despite his addictions, Halsted landed a job in 1886 at what eventually became Baltimore's Johns Hopkins University. There, he joined an eccentric crew that included William Welch, a bachelor known for his love of carnival rides, and William Osler, a Canadian doctor who used alliteration to help students remember things, such as "fingers, food, flies, and filth led to typhoid fever." Osler would also be credited with the saying "A physician who treats himself has a fool for a patient."

At Hopkins, Halsted created new techniques to repair hernias and suture intestines; he invented what became the first surgical glove. But his most important innovation was in how surgeons were trained. Instead of a short apprenticeship, he and his colleagues required surgeons to all but live in the hospital for six to eight years, hence the name *residents*. Residents weren't allowed to marry, were on call 362 days a year, and typically worked more than one hundred hours a week. Through time, practice, and a crushing workload, residents were given more responsibility until their last year, when they had almost complete autonomy, a role handled today by chief residents. Halsted's motto was "See one, do one, teach one." Some of the world's most famous surgeons worked under Halsted and Osler, including Harvey Cushing, the father of neurosurgery. Schools across the world adopted the Hopkins residency model.

A century later, the University of Virginia's neurosurgery department still had the manic values of the old Hopkins program. In Dilan's first week of residency, the department chairman, John Jane, showed him how to do spinal decompressions and herniated discs. Soon, he was doing the procedure alone—and found himself completely lost when he operated on a man who had two prior decompression operations. He opened the patient's neck and was facing a mass of white stuff. *Was it scar tissue or bone or the spinal cord itself?* He asked the nurse to call Dr. Jane.

The nurse turned from the phone. "Dr. Jane said to keep going. He'll be down in a little bit."

He poked around a bit more. If that white material was scar tissue, he could continue. But if he cut the spinal cord, he would paralyze the guy from the neck down. He asked the nurse to call Dr. Jane again.

"Dr. Jane said he's rounding. He'll be down soon."

More minutes passed. He stood over the patient, looked at the open incision.

I can't just stand here and do nothing. He cut deeper, still lost in the clouds of white matter and bone. Then, suddenly, he saw that the scar tissue had a slightly different tone and texture. *So that's the scar tissue, and that's the spinal cord.* He knew *exactly* what to cut, and what not to cut. Now, instead of panic, he felt a wave of confidence flow through his body, a mix of warmth and calmness that he'd never experienced in medical school. In that transformational moment, he thought, *Yes, I have what it takes to be a great neurosurgeon.*

Practice, experience, pressure. Chief residents and attending physicians barked like drill sergeants, backing residents against the wall, spittle forming at the sides of their mouths. You rarely sat in the presence of an attending physician, and if you did, you made sure you were in the back rows. When you walked down the hall with an attending, you did so a step to the side and behind; the attending was the ship, and residents and medical students were the wake. No other way to get good. It's how human brains are wired. New experiences create neural connections. Create enough neural connections and you have a network, a subroutine responsible for a particular action or thought. The connections in these subroutines are like highway systems in a growing city. Activate them over and over, and the myelin casings on the nerve pathways actually grow thicker. It's like adding lanes to a highway, which allows even more traffic to flow through. This is how people learn to drive, concentrating at first on the steering wheel and how it moves the car, and then as the neural connections and muscles become established, doing it without thinking. It's how great basketball players dribble and dunk. It's how surgeons master simple procedures and then move to more complex ones, and then do those with a kind of intuition that borders on art.

Dilan did surgeries when he was sick, on weekends, and early in the morning, 120 hours a week. He was lucky if he had three hours of sleep in his own bed. He'd begun to lose his hair, so he shaved his head. It was all or nothing. One month he was home for just twenty-one hours total. You moved all day and often didn't stop until four in the morning. When he ran out of clean underwear, he cut up scrubs to make new boxer shorts so he wouldn't have to go home and change. It was exhausting but addictive. You fixed people's problems quickly, turned paralysis into movement, removed tumors that caused people blistering headaches. *A chance to cut was a chance to cure.* If you perfected the procedures and got faster, you could help even more people. *Nothing heals like cold, hard steel.*

He was happiest when the operating rooms were like battle zones overflowing with casualties. Some of his peers couldn't hack it. One broke down during a spine operation and ran out of the OR. Another was arrested for beating his girlfriend and eventually committed suicide. A third one nearly choked an emergency department physician. Some residents hallucinated and were so exhausted they slept with their eyes open. He wasn't immune. Sometimes, he and the other residents rested their foreheads against the microscope and fell asleep. A chief resident fell backward once when someone moved the microscope. Dilan's worst fear was that he would fall asleep against the microscope and topple into a patient's open brain. After one sleepless stretch, he came home, grabbed a beer, and collapsed into a rocking chair on the porch. He woke up the next morning, still in the chair, still holding the beer in his right hand, unspilled. Another day, halfway into an incision, he heard his name, as if someone was calling from afar. He looked across the operating table. The nurse's eyes were wide open. He looked down. A No. 10 scalpel was in his right hand; the blade was on the purplish blue line he'd just drawn on the patient's skin, right over the lower back. He finished the incision and placed the knife on a tray.

After the nurses suctioned blood from the incision, he picked up a Bovie, dissected some yellow fatty tissue, then heard that faraway voice again.

"Dr. Ellegala? Are you all right? Dr. Ellegala?"

He shook himself awake again. "Call the attending," he told the nurse. The attending rushed into the room and took over. Dilan stood by the table, his head jerking up and down as he fell asleep and woke himself up.

He went through cases like a circular saw goes through oak—682 neurosurgeries in one year, as far as he knew, more than any other resident in the department's history. In 2003 when medical trade groups issued new rules to limit residents' hours to eighty a week, Dilan rounded up his colleagues. They agreed: the only way to be a great surgeon was to do procedures over and over, thicken those myelin sheaths. As far as Dilan was concerned, it was as if someone said, "No, you can't be a great surgeon." They agreed to ignore the new rules. "No one tells us how to learn," he would say.

So many surgeries. And so much death. During one three-day period, he told nine families that their loved ones were gone. When he broke bad news to families, he watched their eyes fill with tears. Some screamed. Some fainted. Some grew angry. Yes, that chief resident in Seattle was an asshole, but fatigue and death could make anyone numb and a little crazy. He knew because it was happening to him.

The caseload was crushing. Death was everywhere. But you were a rock star, at least within the hospital district. In some ways, this twisted your worldview more than anything else. Neurosurgeons were at the top of the medical pyramid, higher even than heart surgeons; sometimes it seemed all you had to do was hint you were a brain surgeon and you'd get laid. Patients were off-limits, but everyone else in the hospital was fair game. He and other residents found ways to have sex whenever and wherever they could: while a patient was wheeled down the hall for an MRI; in supply closets, stairwells, call rooms. Their bodies might crave sleep, but the male residents still went downtown to South Street Brewery to pick up women. "We few, we happy few, we band of brothers," John Jane would sometimes say, quoting Shakespeare. And he was right. You were a soldier on leave, grabbing what life you could before the next battle. So crazy, so exciting. And afterward, like a hangover, so empty. As the years passed and the failed relationships piled up, he realized that sex was a diversion. Relief from exhaustion. Relief from all the death around him. Like a drug.

He was in his midthirties by then, nearly three decades after that day on the school track in South Dakota, the day he promised his father he'd be a doctor at Harvard, not Yale. And now he was there, doing a cerebrovascular fellowship, goal achieved. He felt the history of the place wrap around him. Harvard Medical School had grand buildings of white Vermont marble in the quadrangle. The old brick Peter Bent Brigham Hospital was behind them, and the new glass and steel towers of the Brigham and Women's Hospital rose into the sky like monuments to medicine's future. Some days between less challenging cases, he slipped out the department's back door and took an alley to Harvard's Countway Library of Medicine. He went to a lower floor where leather-bound journals were kept. He looked for the oldest spines he could find. When he turned pages, paper fragments fell off like bits of tissue. The musty paper smelled like time itself. He looked around, thinking, *I can't believe I'm holding the first editions of* Nature *and the* New England Journal of Medicine.

When he was done, he returned to the Peter Bent Brigham building. He heard the echo of his feet as he climbed two flights of stairs around the building's central rotunda. He passed the white columns and followed the blue metal railing to his office, just a desk crammed between two walls, more like a closet than a room. But the man who once worked behind those walls! Harvey Cushing himself—the doctor who perfected the craniotomy, the workaholic, a surgeon so respected by his peers that they formed a fan club called the Harvey Cushing Society—was a lion. The prototype.

Dilan found Arthur Day an estimable heir to Cushing's legacy. Day had a soft, slightly nasal twang; he had piercing blue eyes framed by semicircular eyebrows; he wore round eyeglasses, which accentuated the circular nature of his eyes. He was quick to curse, especially when you made a mistake or couldn't answer his many questions. He'd grown up on a farm in Red Chute, Louisiana, where he took apart cars and tractors. He had jobs as a mailman and a roughneck on an oil rig before he settled on medicine. Growing up around machines, he developed a consuming desire to understand what made them work and why they failed. If you understood how all the parts fit together, it was a cinch to fix them. But you had to go deep, beyond what you thought you knew. You might know how to unlock a door—just turn the key. But once you studied the shape of the key, its ridges and curves, and how it fit into the keyhole, and how the ridges and curves turned the tumblers, and how the tumblers moved and connected with the deadbolt, then you truly understood how to unlock a door. You might be able to pick it without a key. If you didn't understand the mechanics, you could ruin the mechanism altogether when taking it apart.

The same was true about the brain's anatomy. And because even the smallest mistake could be devastating, perfection was the only reasonable goal. This obsession had served him well as a surgeon, earning him a national reputation in Florida before Harvard recruited him. He did things Dilan thought were impossible.

During one operation Dilan watched Day confront an aneurysm that looked like a snake digesting a rat. Usually a neurosurgeon put a clip on the neck of an aneurysm, but this anaconda had no neck. Instead, Day stacked several curved clips against each other to create a tunnel. The clips weren't supposed to be used that way, but it worked. Another time, Dilan watched Day control a rupturing aneurysm. Patients often died on the table when this happened. Day stomped his feet up and down, as if running in place. As he saved that patient, he said in his Louisiana drawl, "Dilan, save me from myself! Save me from myself!"

Still, as Dilan walked past the old echoing walls of the Peter Bent Brigham building, he saw the same cracks in himself and his profession that he found at Virginia and the University of Washington.

The cracks only grew wider after the cardiac standstill he and Day did early in his fellowship. Dilan had visited the woman every two hours after the operation; he'd done sternal rubs and other tests. By the next day, it was clear that she was gone.

He found Arthur Day in his office the following weekend. Day was on the verge of tears. They went over the case for hours.

Reducing the blood pressure to zero or close to it was standard operating procedure, but Dilan thought that keeping the blood pressure at fifteen made more sense. You would have a greater risk of bleeding, but at least you could see those perforator vessels, a small price for clarity. Before Dilan had a chance to raise the issue, Arthur Day did it himself. "Yeah, maybe we should have left it up a little."

It was too late for that patient, but her death could help someone in the future. Forgive and remember.

But something else had gone wrong, and it had more to do with Dilan than the operation. He recalled his excitement before the operation, how amped up he was about doing something other doctors only read about.

It was all about my ego.

Suddenly it seemed so clear: surgical achievement could be just as addictive as a drug. Like addiction, the quest for surgical success etched new neural subroutines into your brain's circuitry. As this circuitry changed, you changed your life to support this addiction, until you were someone entirely different than you expected or hoped to be. You lost a bit of yourself, your goodness. He'd spent all these years training to be a great surgeon only to find out that this didn't automatically make you a good person. The side effects of this were all around him: doctors who found it easier to talk to residents than their own children, who cheated on their spouses. The neurosurgery department at Harvard was roiling with internal conflicts over pay and favoritism. A female spine surgeon would sue the Brigham and Women's Hospital and Arthur Day, alleging that she was treated differently from male doctors. She would testify that Day told her things like, "You're just a little girl, you know; can you do that spine surgery?" She would allege that Dong Kim, another neurosurgeon, put his arm on her back and said, "Why don't we leave this place and go to the Elliott Hospital so I can give you an oral exam." And later she would testify how a resident threw her into a scrub sink and the garbage. Day and Kim would deny the allegations, but a jury would render a $1.6 million jury verdict against the hospital, and a $20,000 judgment against Day. Both Arthur Day and Dong Kim would eventually leave Harvard for positions in the western United States.

Late one night Dilan was in the rotunda of the old Peter Bent Brigham Hospital when he bumped into Peter Black, the department's chairman. Black's tired eyes suggested that he'd been working since sunup. By then, Dilan had two job offers: one from Oregon Health and Science University in Portland and another from the University of Pittsburgh.

Pittsburgh had a better reputation in neurosurgery circles, but he'd also heard it was similar to the University of Virginia: incredible pressure, lots of sexual intrigue. Peter Black looked down at the marble floor.

"If I were you, I'd go to a place where you can have a life."

Have a life.

There it was again.

He would go to Oregon.

But before he settled in at Oregon, he would take six months off. No matter what it did to his career. He wanted to be a good person and a good teacher, someone who showed students how it felt to drill a hole into a skull, how the skull had layers, how you could feel the density change just before the damn bit broke through. He'd go to Africa to reassess. Colleagues sometimes quoted the French doctor René Leriche, who said, "Every surgeon carries within himself a small cemetery where from time to time he goes to pray." It was time for him to pray, to bring his career to a standstill to see what kind of man he truly wanted to be.

CHAPTER 12

In the passing weeks, Dilan had only partially resisted Oystein Olsen's pleas to take call. The pediatric ward had a chronic staff shortage, so when a group of Tanzanian clinicians left Haydom for a training event, Oystein made another pitch, and this time Dilan said okay. He thought, *At least they're at a legitimate medical meeting; I'm not taking someone's job.* But there amid the crying babies he realized he'd forgotten much of what he'd learned in medical school about pediatrics. *Oh well, I'll go with it.* He played up his incompetence in front of the nurses, especially Angela, the head nurse. "Angela, what do I do?" he said with a pained face when confronted with a virus or malaria case. "I'm just a neurosurgeon; I don't know anything about this stuff!" The nurses giggled and put their hands in front of their mouths. He thought, *Yes, make them feel smarter than a neurosurgeon; give them a shot of confidence; build their morale. That will help more children in the long run.*

And all this came with an added benefit: sneaking out of the ward early. "You've got everything under control, Angela, you don't need me!"

He often took long walks into town. Above him, the bare branches of the jacaranda trees moved in the wind, casting shadow webs on the baked red dirt. The soil stained his brown Keens orange-red. Boys and girls in their teens took hard-packed paths to a community water tank and waited their turns at the spigot. Gusts on the plateau picked up loose soil and sent it spinning. Twisters appeared more frequently because of the dust and sun and wind. The rain should have come by now.

He followed the road back to the hospital compound and poked around the garage, where mechanics wiped dust from their tools and brows. He watched them yank out bearings and bushings and move their grease-stained hands into the ambulances' entrails. Around the corner from the garage, hospital workers piled sheets soiled with blood and feces into great metal vats. The textiles spun in the water, which turned brown and white from the dirt and soap. The hospital didn't have dryers, so workers pulled out the laundry and hung sheets and blankets on lines in a courtyard or placed them on the ground in a patchwork quilt.

As he explored these places, Dilan let his mind go. A nap? Perfect. Books he had denied himself during residency? He cracked open their spines. He found himself paging through his *Lonely Planet*. He thought about the camping trips he might do. He was opening the bellows. Some people might find it strange that he was spending six months at a bush-town hospital to relax. But when you work hundred-hour weeks year after year, doing a few surgeries in the morning and then having afternoons and evenings absolutely free—well, that didn't fit his definition of work.

Jenny was there to work. And she'd flung herself into it. He got it. He would have done exactly the same thing in medical school, prove yourself any way you can.

In Haydom, she returned to the cottage late at night with stories about patients with giant abscesses, oozing pus; patients with broken bones turning yellow because they had been exposed to air for too long. On her second day in the Lena pediatrics ward, she was called to certify the death of a teenage girl who died from malnutrition; the girl's body was still warm when she entered the room; her mother sobbed; other children and parents in the room watched with wide eyes. She didn't have a medical degree, but here she was examining patients, ordering diagnostic tests and treatments, and writing URGENT on paper slips to get results back more quickly. When test results didn't come back fast enough, she did them herself. A typical attending physician in a North American intensive care unit might have ten to twenty patients; here in Haydom, she was in charge of forty. She walked into their cottage at night exhausted but on fire.

He would be on the couch looking way too relaxed. He should be in the wards helping people, she told him. Wasn't saving lives more important than reading a book or goofing off with the mechanics?

"I'm not here just to work," he said over and over.

But that wire saw made it just a bit harder to resist such pressure. And even some of the other foreign doctors were saying he was lazy. The Lena Ward was filled with babies whose heads were enlarged from hydrocephalus. Why not do more?

He thought, *I can fill the next six months with as much surgery as I did in residency. But then what?*

He would leave Africa just as burned-out as he was when he arrived. Nothing inside him would have changed. Nothing around him either. No one would take his place after he left. That wire saw would end up rusty and broken, just like that ancient Gigli saw he'd found in the storage room.

As Jenny pressed, he felt his mind narrow into a blade and touch a deep place, old memories and new ones together now.

Those morning meetings. Medical students sitting? Unthinkable at the University of Virginia, treasonous at Harvard, or most any serious teaching hospital. A violation of the hierarchy, tradition, history; like foot soldiers failing to salute. But here they were in Haydom—medical students, visitors—sitting as if their parents handed them front-row tickets to a Live Aid concert. *What made them think they had a hall pass? Because they were Westerners in Africa?*

He'd seen a similar dynamic in Sri Lanka. When he was a teen, his family returned to visit relatives. Kandy was full of tourists, mostly northern Europeans, strolling around the lake and filing by the Sacred Temple of the Tooth Relic. To him, the visitors' voices were full of condescension and entitlement, as if they were saying, "Look at how quaint and backward these people are."

Worse, the Sri Lankans just seemed to take it. When tourists walked down the street, the Sri Lankans parted like water from a ship's bow. When a Sri Lankan and a tourist went to a restaurant cashier, the cashier took the tourist's money first. *This isn't right. This is Kandy, home of the Sacred Tooth, the kingdom that fought off the Dutch and Portuguese, my home, not theirs.* After a family meal at the

Elephant House restaurant, he walked down the center of the side-walk, straight toward the tourists. He was the ship; they would be the wake. He bumped them if they didn't move.

"*Malli, malli* (little brother, little brother). You should step aside," his cousins had said.

"Why should I? It's not their country."

It's not their country. His mind moved from the morning report to the radiology meeting and then to *Sala*, morning prayers. Same pattern: in the chapel, the foreign doctors typically sat near the front and together, while the Tanzanian nurses, orderlies, and clinical officers sat in the back and to the side, as if they were the visitors. *This isn't right.*

After *Sala* one morning, he crossed the hospital's courtyard on his way to the radiology meeting room. He wore his long, white doctor's coat. Its three buttons were fastened. His head was freshly shaved. His eyes had that eagle look.

He passed through the waiting room. It was full of patients but had a chapel-like hush as he strode down the hall. To his right, a technician hung X-ray films to dry. In the meeting room, he found a spot near the back with the Tanzanian clinical officers. Baba Naman sorted X-rays and paperwork, reading glasses perched on the tip of his nose.

As usual, the visiting students and doctors poured in and sat near the front. His eyes narrowed. Just before Naman spoke, Dilan raised his voice.

"So, since this hospital belongs to the Tanzanians, I think it would be better if the visiting students offered them their seats."

Heads turned. Dilan stood with his feet apart, arms folded, chin up slightly. Another push. "These are the most important people in the room. They're the ones who will be here when we're gone." He waited.

Silence, then the sound of movement: chair legs against the floor, the rustle of clothing, keys and coins in pockets. The students stood, turned, and offered the Tanzanians their seats. The students didn't look put out. Maybe some were relieved; when you travel to another country, it's difficult to decipher its mores. But several Tanzanians waved their hands, as if to say, "It's OK, no problem." The medical students looked at Dilan and then back at the Tanzanians and then insisted. Reshuffled, the room grew quiet. Baba Naman placed an X-ray on the light board.

It's a start.

But, later, he thought, *It wasn't enough. He had made a statement about who was truly important here, but would that really change the dynamics? Probably not. What else can I do?* He could teach the Tanzanian clinicians how to read CT scans and X-rays of the brain, but this meant teaching them about conditions they couldn't heal—lessons in frustration.

But what if he taught someone how to fix those problems?

It would have to be basic stuff: biopsies, abscesses, craniotomies, hematomas. After his six months were up, a Tanzanian could take over. A Tanzanian could save lives instead of a *mzungu*. That wire saw wouldn't end up in the storage room, rusting. *That would have true impact.*

The idea generated momentum in his mind until it seemed so obvious: "See one, do one, teach one," Halsted had said. You could go back even further. The Latin root for *doctor* wasn't *healer*. It was *teacher.*

He turned it over in his mind that night. Was it arrogant of him to think he could teach someone brain surgery without any consultation from the Tanzanian government? Was he any better than those foreign medical students who thought they could do things differently in Africa . . . because they were in Africa?

Yes, it was arrogant, absolutely, he thought. But there was a difference. The arrogance of the foreign medical students perpetuated the status quo—the idea that visitors were in charge. His arrogance was designed to change the status quo, to send a message to

Tanzanians that they could take care of their own people. Foreigners were just that: visitors here to assist. His goal was to empower instead of oppress.

But, is it right to teach someone with such little formal medical education? After all, Mayegga had the American equivalent of a high school education and a few years of clinical training. If a doctor in North America suddenly pulled a paramedic or physician assistant aside for a brain surgery lesson, said doctor might be sued into oblivion—maybe put in jail if a patient ended up harmed.

But what's the alternative?

The reality on the ground was that millions of people had no access to even the most basic forms of neurosurgery. If you required equivalent standards of care, then you were consigned to doing nothing at all. Was that right? Was it ethical to wait until a country built a stable of experienced surgeons, a process that might take decades, if it could happen at all? Or should you continue to depend on teams of visiting neurosurgeons, which would never fill the demand? Didn't that just perpetuate the status quo?

Standing by is not acceptable, he thought. Besides, teaching surgery always involved a truth that both patients and doctors didn't always like to think about: the conflict between a patient's best interest and society's. Patients rightly want the best surgeon available. But hospitals, and by extension, future patients, must have a steady supply of new surgeons. This means you would always have hospitals where inexperienced hands cut someone's flesh. Western teaching hospitals dealt with this tension by creating layers of backup: chief residents watched junior ones, and overseeing it all were attending doctors. It was an imperfect system—if your mother needed her gallbladder taken out, would you really want a junior resident holding the scalpel? But it also had produced the world's best surgeons.

He made his decision. He would teach someone basic brain surgery. Like an attending physician in a Western hospital, he would be the student's backup here. *Anything he fucks up, I can fix.*

But who should he teach? He couldn't force this on someone. It had to be a special person. He had an idea of who that might be.

CHAPTER 13

Next morning, every seat in the radiology meeting was taken. A few visiting medical students had gotten the message and stood in the rear, but others still settled in the front. Dilan asked them again to move. "None of you will be here in a few months," he said, trying to keep his voice light and friendly. Inside, he seethed.

Naman finished with the X-rays and lowered a projection screen to go over the CT scans.

"We have a twenty-three-year-old woman, sudden onset of unconsciousness." Naman turned around.

"Dr. Dilan, what do you think of this scan? What should we do with this patient?"

Long pause.

"So, I could answer that question, but I think that's not the right thing to do. It's not right because I could come here and treat all the neurosurgical patients myself, but I'm leaving. What happens to these patients when I'm gone? Who will take care of them?"

He scanned the room and found Emmanuel Mayegga.

He'd been watching how Mayegga handled himself around patients and staff. Mayegga was an assistant medical officer, which meant he had a few more years of training than clinical officers. More important, he carried himself differently from the other clinicians. He walked a little taller, spoke a little louder. In Dilan's experience, you could walk into a room full of doctors and pick out the surgeons merely by observing their body language. He'd found that many surgeons leaned forward when they spoke, held people a little longer with their eyes. Surgeons had a bit of a swagger. Mayegga had that swagger.

"So, Dr. Mayegga, what do you think of this CT scan? What would you do with this patient?" He made a point of calling him Dr. Mayegga, even though he was just a clinician.

"Well, I'm not a neurosurgeon. How can I know?"

"When I leave, what will you do with patients like her? Send them home or wait for me or someone else to come and treat your people?"

"I don't know how to treat this woman. I'm not a neurosurgeon."

"You could be a neurosurgeon. And if you were, then you'd be able to take care of your own people."

"But I'm not a neurosurgeon."

Mayegga's eyes darted back and forth as if searching for more words. Dilan backed off. He'd made his point. But had he gone too far?

When the meeting broke up, Dilan went straight to Mayegga and offered his hand.

"Hey, man, I apologize. I didn't mean to put you on the spot."

"It is not a problem," Mayegga said.

"But I still think it's unacceptable how the foreign doctors come here and take over."

"I agree, but what is there to do?"

"Well, I meant it when I said that you can learn this stuff. I can teach you how to read brain scans. Let's go over some tonight. You can learn this."

Mayegga glanced at Baba Naman, who was standing nearby, listening.

"You should try," Naman said.

They met at dusk back in the meeting room. Baba Naman sat at his desk, organizing requests for X-rays and CT scans and getting ready for Mayegga's first brain anatomy lesson. Dilan and Mayegga sat next to him as Naman called up the first scan.

"Dr. Mayegga," Dilan said, "tomorrow, I'm going to ask you to diagnose several brain conditions. It will look like I'm asking you out of the blue. But then you'll answer the questions as if you've always known about the brain and CT scans. Everyone will wonder what's going on. This will be the first step in you becoming a neurosurgeon."

Mayegga shook his head.

"I don't know, I don't know. Is this possible?"

"Absolutely. I'll give you the answers tonight!"

He turned toward the image on Naman's computer monitor: a black-and-white scan of a brain. It was shaped like a giant almond with a centerline dividing the hemispheres.

"When I look at a CT, my first question is always 'Is what I'm looking at abnormal or normal?' Then my next question is always: 'Why?'"

Their heads moved closer as they studied the image.

"This image is normal, and here's how you can tell. Look first around the edges." He traced his finger around the white oval-shaped line of the skull. "Is there something that's pushing the brain in some way? In this case, no. Then you look at the ventricles."

On the CT scan, the ventricles spread out like two butterfly wings.

"That's where the spinal fluid is made and held. Now look at the midline."

Dilan pointed toward a white line that divided the right and left hemispheres. "It's straight and hasn't shifted right or left, which means nothing is pushing or pulling on it. Everything is where it should be. So, Dr. Mayegga. Is this a normal brain?"

Mayegga studied the image.

"Normal," he said.

"Why is it normal?"

Mayegga explained. The edges around the brain looked even, a nicely rounded oval; no opening in the skull or a tumor that made the skull bulge; the midline looked straight.

"Excellent!"

Naman called up another scan, one of a child with hydrocephalus. The image showed the misshapen cranium; the ventricles were distorted from the pressure.

"Normal or abnormal?"

"Abnormal."

"Yes, and tomorrow, I'm going to ask you the same question, and when I ask, 'Why?,' you'll say the ventricles are big, and that's abnormal."

Mayegga smiled nervously.

"So, Dr. Mayegga, is this abnormal or normal?"

"Abnormal?"

"Exactly! Why?"

The wind blew hard all night. Something outside the cottage made a clanking noise that woke Dilan and reminded him of the thin foam mattress underneath him. The coffee barely cut through his mind's haze. It was still blowing as foreign doctors and clinical officers hustled toward Radiology. Gusts wrapped their white coats tightly around them, then at other times ripped them open and made them fly like flags. Dilan noticed some of the women trying to fix their hair. A shaved head had its benefits.

He was as unsettled as the wind. They'd spent hours going over scans the night before. Dilan had taught Mayegga how the midline curved when someone's head was struck, how fluid could build in the ventricles at the center of the brain. He showed him the differences between a tumor and an abscess. Hyperdense areas were bright white and could be an intraparenchymal hemorrhage, a head injury. Hypodense areas were darker and could mean someone had an infection or ischemia. Mayegga seemed to have a blade-sharp memory, but how would he do the next day?

Mayegga was a tough read. One moment he was cocky, the next he scrunched up his eyes and furrowed his brows in what looked like anger. Maybe it was just his way of concentrating. Then his face opened and his eyes sparkled in almost childlike insecurity. Dilan didn't want to embarrass the guy. That could do more harm than good. That could kill something inside Mayegga and maybe the other Tanzanians as well.

This was more than just a silly trick. He had just six months here. Turning Mayegga into a brain surgeon would require some rewiring: first and foremost, Mayegga would have to truly believe he could operate on the human brain. It was a subtle change. Mayegga would need to gain the confidence Dilan had found when John Jane left him alone in that spinal decompression operation so many years ago. Medical schools eased their students through this process with books, rotations, and time, none of which Dilan could provide. Without this mind shift, Mayegga wouldn't even consider learning brain surgery. Dilan would have to look for other candidates.

But he could help Mayegga through this door by changing the context, in this case, how other doctors perceived him, foreign and Tanzanian alike. If Mayegga fooled everyone about his knowledge of the brain's anatomy, then he would suddenly experience what it's like to be a brain surgeon; the looks of admiration, the raised eyebrows, the respect. That burst of recognition from others would serve as fuel. In the coming weeks, they would go over one CT scan after another. Mayegga would need that external motivation to push through his insecurities, open his mind to things he never thought possible.

When Mayegga entered the radiology room, Dilan nodded, as if to say, "You're on." Dilan took a spot in the rear, as usual. Mayegga went to the middle and took a seat.

"Now, here are some CTs to do," Baba Naman announced in a theatrical way. "A neurosurgeon is here, and so Dr. Dilan, could we please go through these?"

Dilan folded his arms. "Please, Dr. Mayegga. Come to the front and show us what you are seeing."

People swiveled in their seats, first toward Dilan and then Mayegga.

Naman handed a wooden pointer stick to another Tanzanian clinician, who handed it to Mayegga. Dilan noticed some of the Tanzanians chuckle when Naman did this. Passing the stick seemed to have some symbolic meaning that he didn't quite understand. A few of the European doctors wrinkled their brows.

"So, Dr. Mayegga, for those in the audience who haven't looked at CT scans, this area over here, the darker area, what do you see?"

Mayegga described how cerebrospinal fluid could build inside someone's brain.

"So what is your diagnosis?"

"Hydrocephalus."

"Yes, exactly!"

The foreign doctors glanced at each other. Other than radiologists and neurologists, most doctors don't know much about brain scans. And here was Mayegga, a non-MD, teaching them.

Naman put up another image.

Dilan said, "Can you show the medical students and the others why this is abnormal?"

Mayegga said, "This is a CT scan with contrast. You can tell this because the fatty tissue around the eyes is lighter. That is a sign of contrast."

He pointed toward a dark gray blob.

"That means this mass that you see here in the front is not a tumor."

"How do you know it's not a tumor?" Dilan asked, businesslike. "Can you educate the rest of us who don't know?"

"A tumor has blood vessels that are leaky, and the contrast can cross the blood-brain barrier. If it is a tumor, then the contrast will go inside the tumor, and it will look white. It means it is enhancing. But the mass is dark. If it is a dark mass in the center, it is more likely to be an abscess."

"Exactly!"

He looked at Mayegga, who stood calm and straight, arms crossed. He detected a hint of a smile. He glanced at the medical students and saw nods of respect. He turned toward the Tanzanian clinicians, whose eyes were a little wider than usual. At that moment, he felt something shift in the room. For once, it felt equal.

After the performance, Dilan rushed over to Mayegga, shook his hand, and put his other hand on Mayegga's shoulder.

"Now, that was impressive. That's how it's done. You were perfect."

Mayegga beamed.

Time to double down. Dilan was headed to the theater to do a craniotomy with the wire saw.

"So, do you want to do it with me?"

"But I'm not really a neurosurgeon."

"Sure you are. Look how well you did today."

From a purely technical standpoint, many brain surgeries aren't that difficult. What's different are the stakes. Damage a small piece of the liver, and it will regenerate. Slice the skin and it heals. Once you cut the wrong thing inside the brain, it's often cut for good. A neurosurgeon named Frank Vertosick Jr. once compared it to walking on a foot-wide plank. Put the plank on a driveway, and you would have no problem walking on it without falling. But you experience that same plank differently if it was suspended ten stories in the air.

Mayegga hesitated. "I don't know if this is a good idea. I am not trained."

"I'll train you. You can do anything, man. And why would you let foreigners like me come in and take care of your people? I'll be leaving anyway. You should be doing it."

"I could get in trouble."

"Don't worry. I won't let that happen." *Anything he fucks up I can fix.*

But first he'd have to see Mayegga's reaction to a living brain. They had a term for doctors who freaked out during brain surgery: "peek and shriek."

Some neurosurgeons might expose the brain, see the risks, and close as fast as they could, as if opening a closet and seeing a ghost—peek and shriek. Often, they told patients the problem was inoperable, which as far as Dilan was concerned, was a lie to cover up their fear or lack of experience. What would Mayegga do when he saw an exposed brain?

They sorted through green scrubs and washed their hands in the sink in the hallway. They donned caps and masks and went into the theater. The patient was on the table.

"Let's close the door, please," Dilan said. The nurses often left it open, a vector for infections and flies.

He shaved the patient's head, doused it with iodine, and made an incision. He explained each step as he did them. He retracted the scalp, exposing the skull. He took the Hudson Brace drill and rotated the handle. He waited for the click. Somewhere burned in his mind was the memory of how he had drilled into a woman's brain. Time to make amends.

"Dr. Mayegga, you can feel different layers of the bone as you go through. You can feel the click as it stops. You want pressure but not too much."

He cranked until it clicked, and he wiped away the bone dust. He made another hole. He picked up the wire saw and slipped it into one hole and out the other. He moved it back and forth and cut through the skull. He cut off a patch and exposed the dura mater, the brain's outermost membrane.

"This is the dura. Touch it. You can feel the thickness."

Mayegga pressed his finger on the dura, the outermost layer of the meninges, felt its fibrous, leathery texture.

"In Latin, *dura mater* means 'tough mother.' Now what you want to do is cut it. Let me show you."

He grabbed a sharper No. 11 scalpel and cut the dura.

"You'll see it's really a couple of layers. Just underneath is the arachnoid—a thinner layer with fibers like a spiderweb. And underneath that layer is the pia." He pointed to the pia's translucent film, an impermeable barrier between the meninges and the brain. When the pia becomes irritated, the brain develops meningitis, a common affliction in Haydom. From now on, Mayegga would be able to visualize what was happening inside the heads of his meningitis patients.

"Now if you cut too deeply, your patient will be paralyzed or have a stroke and will never recover." You can concentrate so hard on a piece of anatomy that you forget the stakes, that this mass of pink and pulsating tissue in front of you contains everything a person is and hopes to be.

He handed Mayegga the scalpel, then took his hand and showed him how to hold it.

Mayegga looked up, his eyes wide, questioning.

"Go for it."

Mayegga positioned the scalpel and cut the dura.

"Perfect."

Dilan took over, peeling back the triangular flap, exposing the brain's cauliflower-like folds. It was pink, and it pulsed.

Dilan raised his voice so everyone in the room could hear him clearly.

"OK, Dr. Mayegga, this is the living human brain. Take your pointing finger and wet it a little. You don't want it to stick."

Mayegga glanced at him. Dilan nodded to go ahead.

Mayegga put some saline on his finger, and Dilan took his hand. Dilan guided his finger toward the patient's brain and then into it.

"Whoa! Not so hard, not so hard!"

Mayegga's hand flinched back as if he'd touched a hot poker. Dilan laughed.

"I'm just messing with you."

Mayegga was slow to put his finger forward so Dilan guided his hand again, pressing harder than Mayegga expected.

"It's OK, you can use this much pressure."

Then Dilan released his hand so Mayegga could touch it on his own. Mayegga pressed, and then pressed in a different place.

Good. He's taking his time. He's not intimidated. He's exploring. He's got the balls. Now, loudly, loud enough for people in the hallway to hear:

"Today, Dr. Mayegga, you're touching the living human brain. How many other people in the world can say that?"

CHAPTER 15

At dusk Emmanuel Mayegga passed through the hospital gates and turned toward Haydom town. The dust was thick at this intersection, especially when the hospital's ambulances rumbled through. As the dust swirled, men covered their mouths and noses with their *shuka* blankets, but Mayegga wore Western clothes—leather shoes, trousers, and a shirt with a collar, nothing to filter the particles from his lungs. He thought, *This new* mzungu *could get me in trouble.*

Mayegga was Iraqw, a group thought to have migrated to the Mbulu Highlands from what today is Ethiopia and Somalia. Like many Iraqw, he had long arms with thin wrists. His fingers were long and slender. On occasion, a visitor might ask his age, and he'd answer with a shrug and a tenor voice that rose in a good-natured way and then flattened like the plateau below the hospital. "Nobody is very sure. We can only guess."

Then he smiled as if to tell a secret: when you start from zero, why would you need a birthday? And then he told them he was probably born sometime in 1968, and as was common here, he merely picked a date to put on government forms. This put him in his late thirties now, married to Samwayma, a nurse with a hearty laugh, who bore him a son named Godwin, because God always wins.

I'm not a neurosurgeon. But he is so encouraging.

Mayegga knew the roads and paths around Haydom as well as he knew the smile lines on his wife's face, so without thinking, he followed the hospital's barbed-wire fence. Another right turn led down a hill to a building painted in the same beige and red tones as the hospital, Mama Naman's restaurant, Ikunda, the Chagga word for *love.*

The gate was made of wood sticks and a corrugated metal panel. As he had for more than a decade, he walked through it and into a compound that resembled a small *boma*. To his right were three round tables, each with umbrellas made of thatch. Above in a tree, yellow little weaver birds had spun conical nests. He passed a smaller structure made of mud bricks where Mama Naman tended a cook fire.

The bar was at the other end of the courtyard, past a pool table with an uneven slate. A back door led to a patio made of cement that was painted Haydom red. He sat in a red plastic chair, and a waitress brought him a Kilimanjaro beer. If he shifted his seat just right, he could see a tall eucalyptus tree, and then far beyond it, a white rock mountain, a white smudge on the horizon growing gray as the sun set. *The brain pulsated. And it was soft like porridge. Is it possible that I could do neurosurgery?*

The *mzungu* had caused his mind to spin. Then again, the second Dr. Olsen had done the same thing, and look at what happened: he had become a medical officer, respected; making a decent income, enough for a small house in town with four rooms, a metal roof, and a polished floor. That was something, wasn't it?

Baba Naman would join him soon. Naman knew where he began, and how far he'd come. He drank a beer, and the white mountains on the horizon merged with the darkness, gone now, but he could travel there at any time in his mind. Doing so helped put the day's questions in perspective. So, though the horizon had vanished, his mind moved toward it anyway, backward to zero and a time when zero was everything.

First memories were blurry but began on rocks.

Smooth and elephant gray, the rocks were in the hills above the huts, surrounded by brush that hid scorpions and snakes. On the plain below, two oblong boulders rose from the ground like giant heads. The gray boulders and yellow brush mirrored the rainy-season sky, when the sun sent yellow shards through clouds the color of bruises.

One day, when he was perhaps two or three, young Emmanuel was with his mother collecting firewood in the hills above the huts. Suddenly she was gone.

"*Ayi ama?*" he said in Iraqw. Where's *mama?*

He was surrounded by boulders; the *boma* was somewhere below, the fence of brush and thorns that kept out the leopards and hyenas. He cried out again.

"*Ama?*"

Sitting with Baba Naman this evening, he couldn't say how he got back to the safety of the *boma*. Maybe his *mama* found him; maybe some man heard his cry and snatched him before the hyenas did. From time and such distance, memories can mix with dreams.

And then another memory, or was it a dream? They had lived in a hut made of sticks and mud, one room for the animals, the other for his brothers and sisters. The hut had a flat roof made of earth. Inside, wood smoke mingled with earth and animal scents. Timbers were black with soot from the cook fire. He was perhaps four or five, and his mother was gone.

"*Ayi ama?*"

She was gone forever, his father said.

"*Ayi ama?*" He asked anyway because he was stubborn and because it wasn't a dream. His father's second wife would be his *mama* now.

Then, more pain, but this was in his stomach instead of his heart. No rain for months; no water in those boulder dimples; he had to walk for miles to find a water hole. The wind whistled through bare thorn trees. He and his family felt like dry sticks. When the rains finally returned, the sky opened up as if to make up for lost time; torrents fell across the hills and poured through their fields, taking seeds and crops.

They still had a few cattle and goats, so they took arrowheads and slit veins on the necks of the animals, collecting enough blood to fill a small pot but not so much that the animals died. They cooked the blood until it coagulated. It tasted bad, but it was better than the bitter leaves they picked from trees and cooked into mush.

At night he slept on a cattle hide, except when it rained. The water ran thick off the boulder-packed hills above the *boma*, with muddy rivulets flowing down and through the huts. On these wet nights, he assembled rows of small sticks on the ground so the water ran underneath him. He slept on the sticks and used the cattle hide to shield him from the leaks in the flat mud roof.

As he grew older, he hunted tiny dik-dik antelope and sometimes brought down an impala with a poisoned arrow. Dik-diks were smaller and not so smart. He trapped them with sisal ropes. Sometimes, he and other boys scared dik-diks into places between the boulders and killed them with spears and arrows.

Carrying a long stick, he herded the family's goats into the same rocky hills where he once was lost. His world had expanded; now he knew every hill and overhang, even a secret place under a massive boulder with old red rock paintings. Ancient peoples had painted ostriches, giraffes, hippos, and elephants, and while some of those animals could still be found around the *boma*, most had run off as more people trickled into this part of the bush. Not all the drawings were of animals. On a separate rock, an artist had painted a child, arms reaching for a mother, and the mother reaching for the child.

One afternoon on a hill not far from these paintings, he heard a noise.

"Yeaahhn. Yeaahhn."

Sounded like one of his family's goats, but something was off.

He peered around a boulder and saw a python slithering toward him. It was the biggest snake he'd ever seen, maybe fifteen feet long or more. And it was making that same goat-like *yeaahhn*.

He bolted down the mountain, hopping from one rock to another, the snake in pursuit. He didn't stop until he reached the *boma*. Out of breath, he told his father what happened. And, no, he wouldn't go back to collect the goats.

His father laughed. His son was a tough boy, the youngest of his nine children, stubborn, always active, always hunting for something to do, always asking questions. Why this? Why that? Always digging into the ground, and usually so fearless! He wasn't lazy, so his father went after the goats himself, no problem.

Another memory: over the years, enough people had moved to the valley below the boulders that the government opened a primary school. For the first time in his life, he needed money—money for uniforms, school supplies, fees.

So, he trudged for twenty kilometers across the plain to a place below a large mass of white rocks where he found clay. He mined as much as he could carry on his back and hauled it back to the *boma*. He formed the clay into pots and burned them until they were hard. He loaded them on his back, five at a time. He marched to a village thirty kilometers away and sold them for a few shillings.

He worked hard in school and learned Swahili, the national language. He was a quick study. While many older kids returned to their families' *bomas*, his teachers urged him to go to secondary school. The school was close to Dongobesh, too far for daily trips from the *boma*, so he moved in with a relative closer to town, though it was still about six kilometers away. To get to school in time for the 7:15 bell, he woke up before the roosters crowed and ran with his books bouncing on his back. When school was over, he ran home and studied late into the night by a kerosene lamp. He read until he passed out from exhaustion. Sometimes he woke up with his nostrils caked with oily soot.

Secondary school was in English, so he carried a Swahili-to-English dictionary wherever he went, even in the bush while herding goats. He sold more charcoal, more pots, and sometimes he exchanged pots for maize to make homemade beer. As he grew taller and advanced from grade to grade, he told himself, *If you aim for something, there is always a way to hit your mark.*

And now, twenty years later, he was an assistant medical officer, sitting here in Haydom—the horizon of his youth. The second Dr. Olsen, Oystein's father, had opened the door. He'd heard about Mayegga's good marks in secondary school. One day Olsen used the hospital radio channel to summon a pastor, who told some schoolchildren, who told some people who lived near Mayegga's family, who told Mayegga, "Please come to Haydom."

By foot, Haydom was about forty kilometers away. If you started running at sunrise, you might make it there by midday. He left his family's *boma* and ran across the plateau, past acacia trees with their thorny branches in an upward tilt, and an occasional baobab. Near Haydom, the soil changed color, from gray-brown to brownish red.

At the hospital Dr. Olsen looked him up and down. "You should become a clinical officer."

Mayegga wasn't sure what to say. How could he afford such a thing?

But Olsen said the hospital would sponsor him, as long as he returned to Haydom.

A clinical officer?

Mayegga had never imagined such a possibility. But, when a door opens, whether by your hand or another's, you walk through.

For the next three years, he went to clinical officer school in Mwanza, a sprawling city on the shores of Lake Victoria. He studied basic anatomy. He learned to diagnose diseases and prescribe medicines for malaria and tuberculosis. And then he returned to Haydom and learned basic surgical procedures from Dr. Olsen.

The operations were easy enough. His hands had slit the veins of goats to collect blood; his fingers had braided sisal ropes. Was that so different from sorting through muscles and tissues to fix a hernia? He was so proficient that the hospital sent him for two more years of training to become an assistant medical officer, a step above the clinicians who typically worked in small dispensaries. He learned to deliver babies and do Caesareans.

When he returned to Haydom, nurses noticed his speed in the theater, especially Samwayma. He could be demanding and impatient, but she had fallen in love. And he certainly wasn't as rough as some of the European surgeons, who occasionally puffed over things that didn't work or go their way.

Mayegga watched the *mzungu* doctors come and go like those dry-season twisters in the valley. They arrived with eager eyes and safari shirts, their heads spinning with ideas of how things could be done better. They treated a few patients and vanished along with their ideas and plans, then reappeared with different names and faces and more ideas. After a while, they became just another part of the landscape, something to watch for a moment but pay little heed while you did your own work.

And there was plenty to do. Every day on average, the hospital and its outreach clinics treated nine hundred people. Once, a woman came to him after four miscarriages. She had no children yet and feared she would be forever childless, which among the Iraqw was a source of shame. Was she cursed? No, Mayegga had said, he could fix the problem. He tied a strong suture around her cervix to support the fetus. "You must return before you go into labor," he told her. He would remove the suture then and deliver the baby. "If you don't come on time, you and your baby could die."

And the woman had done what he asked; she was at the hospital when it was the baby's time. The *mama* was so happy that she named her new son Mayegga.

Then after so many years of clinical work, he had a thought about his own *mama*. He knew so little about her. Maybe the hospital had records about his *mama*'s death.

He went to the records department and pulled out clothbound ledgers. The pages were yellow-gray and frayed. He scanned the handwritten names and dates until he found her name, Lulu Yahai, and a red cross. She'd died the twenty-fifth of February 1972. Cause of death, cerebral malaria. Certified by the second Dr. Olsen.

Cerebral malaria? A horrible way to go. Normal malaria was bad enough. About three hundred million people around the globe get it every year—he'd probably had malaria himself many times as a child. But roughly one out of a hundred people developed its cerebral form, usually children under the age of five. It hit with the power of a black mamba. Within hours, his *mama* likely would have had convulsions. She would have been in incredible pain. She would have become dizzy and then delirious and eventually fallen unconscious. He'd seen it happen over and over. Closing the ledger, he returned to patients he could save.

Now, at Mama Naman's restaurant, lights from the bar poured through the back door onto the patio, casting Mayegga in half-light. The cement slab of patio dropped sharply to the dirt below. Dr. Dilan had shown him how to use the Hudson Brace to drill into a patient's skull. He'd taken his hand as he cranked and shown how the outer part of the skull felt hard and then softer the deeper the bit went in. He'd shown him the proper pressure so the drill bit didn't suddenly break through. *I think I can learn some things from Dr. Dilan.*

He finished his beer. It was time to go home to Samwayma and Godwin and the hope of more children. His father, Dawita, lived with him now, as well as a brother. The family's center of gravity had shifted away from the *boma* by the boulders toward Haydom, toward him.

Through the back door, he could hear the television. Naman typically set it to news channels, particularly when the country's new president, Jakaya Kikwete, gave a speech.

Mayegga also kept up with news from East Africa, Europe, and the Americas—places far beyond any horizon he could see from Haydom or the boulders of his childhood. He stood and left the flickering images behind, walking into the darkness beyond the patio. What was a horizon, anyway? It's not fixed to one spot; it moves with you, just as the moon moves as you walk out of Mama Naman's restaurant and take the hill toward home.

CHAPTER 16

In the Lena Ward, a two-year-old girl lay in bed, a maroon blanket swaddling her body, her enormous head looking as if it couldn't take another moment of pressure. Fluid had built up inside her skull for months, maybe longer. Still soft because of her age, her skull was shaped like continental Africa, narrow at the base and larger at the top. The pressure had forced her eyes into a downward gaze, which was known as the setting sun phenomenon. Dilan and Mayegga examined her and checked her chart. She'd been vomiting, a sign that her short life was about to set as well.

The human brain forms quickly after conception. It begins as a layer of cells in the embryo, like a blank sheet of paper. Within days the edges of this layer curl toward each other until they close like a scroll. This scroll is now the neural tube. The brain grows at the top of the tube, and the rest becomes the spinal cord. Directed by the baby's DNA, this process happens in about twenty-eight days.

Any number of things can go wrong during and after this process. In about one out of every 2,500 pregnancies, the vertebrae don't line up properly. When this happens, the nerves and meninges slip through and create a sac on the baby's back, a condition called spina bifida.

And in one out of every five hundred births a growing brain fails to develop proper passages for the cerebrospinal fluid to drain. Fluid builds up inside the skull, a condition colloquially called "water on the brain," or hydrocephalus.

Hydrocephalus affects people differently depending on their ages. Older people's skulls don't expand, and the fluid can wreak all sorts of havoc, from headaches to dementia to death if nothing is done. Children under two still have gaps in their skulls called fontanelles, better known as "soft spots." The fontanelles are as thick as canvas and expand as the baby grows. When a child has hydrocephalus, the fluid causes these gaps to stretch even more, which is how babies develop such large heads.

Adults can develop hydrocephalus from head injuries, tumors, and meningitis. In children, infections and traumas during birth are common causes. It's an international problem: in the United States alone, hydrocephalus-related problems cost patients and their insurers $1.4 billion a year. But low-income countries have higher prevalence rates, probably because of untreated infections. Every year in sub-Saharan Africa, more than forty-five thousand babies develop hydrocephalus. Many of these babies' parents have little or no access to doctors. Some take their babies to traditional healers who sear flat metal nails to the babies' big foreheads. A traditional healer might tell parents their babies are cursed and slather the children with the blood of freshly slaughtered chickens.

Surgeons can relieve the pressure by redoing the brain's plumbing. They do this by inserting a tube into the brain. The tube shunts excess spinal fluid into another tube, which carries the fluid into the abdomen where it is absorbed. The tube is called a ventriculoperitoneal shunt, or VP shunt. Few clinics and hospitals in East Africa have the surgeons or equipment to do VP shunt operations. In Haydom, the hospital sometimes referred hydrocephalus patients to the national hospital in Dar es Salaam or hospitals in Arusha and Moshi. Most parents couldn't afford such journeys and took their children home to die.

In Dilan's mind, inserting a VP shunt was a simple operation—much less complicated than a subdural hematoma and light years easier than an aneurysm. North American surgeons typically did them in an hour. He could do them in thirty minutes. It was a good procedure for beginners and perfect for Mayegga. If he could master just this procedure, he would have a huge impact in Haydom. Perfect—if the hospital had any VP shunts to insert.

A shunt is made of three basic parts: a catheter that goes into the ventricles, a valve, and a longer tube to drain fluid away. Dilan and Mayegga looked through the storerooms for some shunts. Maybe a visiting doctor had brought some and stuffed them in a cupboard. None were to be found, and they weren't surprised. *Why would you need shunts if you didn't have a neurosurgeon?* Dilan asked himself.

It might take months to get shunts to Haydom, which wouldn't help the two-year-old in Lena Ward. Was there anything else they could use? He remembered a case at the University of Virginia, a girl with a particularly severe case of hydrocephalus. The fluid had built up so fast that normal shunts couldn't keep up. A typical shunt had a bore of about four millimeters, roughly the diameter of a cocktail straw. The girl needed a bigger tube. So Dilan and his team rifled through a surgical supply closet for something that might work. They found some red catheters with a bore the size of a milk-shake straw. They used it instead of a regular shunt, and the girl did well.

As he and Mayegga looked through the closets, he saw plenty of IV tubing. Would that work?

He found a computer on the second floor of the hospital administration building. The computer's Internet speed was painfully slow, but a study from the 1970s finally appeared on the screen. It discussed the use of IV tubes in extreme cases. *Extreme cases?* Unless they did something soon, the little girl in the Lena Ward would die in excruciating pain. *Time is brain.*

Back in their cottage, Jenny faced Dilan. "Was this what you consider a good outcome?"

Just before they operated on the two-year-old, Dilan and Mayegga worked together on an elderly man with a head injury. They had drilled three burr holes to relieve the pressure. But afterward, the man developed horrific bed sores and a brain abscess. The operation probably caused the abscess to form, and the bedsores erupted because nurses failed to reposition the man's body afterward. The man survived but had to undergo another procedure to drain the abscess. He was in incredible pain.

"Yes, it was a good outcome," Dilan fired back.

Not for the patient, of course. Mayegga had failed to prevent the infection, and worst of all, failed to make sure the hospital staff turned the man in his bed. But all good doctors could trace their successes to moments where they failed. He could talk to Mayegga for hours about proper infection-control techniques, but unless Mayegga experienced the pain of failure—saw with his own eyes how his actions or lack of actions caused needless suffering, well, he would never truly learn. Hit the enemy hard and fast, and deal with the casualties up front. In Mayegga's case, the enemy was time. Once Dilan was gone, Mayegga wouldn't have any backup. The more you babied trainees, the longer you delayed their independence.

They had better success with the makeshift VP shunts. Dilan had shown Mayegga how to drill a hole on the side of the child's head. He'd guided Mayegga's hands as he inserted the IV tube into the ventricles. He'd taught him how to work the rest of the IV tube under the skin down the child's neck and chest until it reached the abdomen. They had operated on the two-year-old girl and several other babies, and they seemed to do well afterward.

Day after day they worked on patients. He taught Mayegga how to use the wire saw to do craniotomies. They did more hydrocephalus cases. They worked on babies and elderly men and women. They talked about each patient afterward—what went right and what went wrong.

As the weeks passed Dilan backed away from the operating table just a tad, another technique to instill confidence. An operating room had invisible zones: one immediately around the patient where the surgeon and scrub nurse worked, and a second ring a few inches outside for students who assisted, and then farther out, a third for observers. If an attending was in your zone, you knew you had backup. If the attending was outside this zone, even just a few steps, you felt as if you were on a high wire.

As Mayegga mastered certain techniques, Dilan stepped out of the first zone. And then as the weeks passed, he stepped from the second to the third, even left the room altogether, peeking through the door now and then to make sure everything was OK. Mayegga needed to know that he would be on his own soon.

But Jenny pressed, "Does he really want to learn?" She asked in a way that told him she was really saying, "It's about your ego, isn't it?"

"That's what I do," Dilan snapped back. "I make neurosurgeons."

In quiet moments, he thought, yes, she made good points. She was a philosophy major in college, after all. And she'd been right before.

During his residency rotation in New Zealand, he had taken a week off to explore the Yasawa Islands off Fiji. The islands were reachable by boat or seaplane and had no doctors. And Fiji itself was short of physicians. Hospitals there sometimes closed because of the lack of anesthesiologists. The entire country had just a handful of surgeons and no neurosurgeons at all. Teams of visiting doctors from Australia and the United States flew in for a week or two, did what they could, and left. When Dilan arrived, word spread quickly that a doctor was on the island. A villager asked shyly if he would see some patients. "Sure," Dilan had replied, not knowing what to expect.

An older man arrived with an abscess boring into his skull. Left untreated, it could eat into his brain. Dilan lanced and cleaned it. He helped a woman with a gynecological issue and treated other villagers' cuts and wounds. The line grew longer. A boy of about eight came with his foot wrapped. He'd cut it on a piece of coral. A traditional healer had packed the wound with leaves and mud. When Dilan removed the bandage, he saw that an infection had eaten away half of the foot. Quickly, Dilan and another villager found a boat and raced across a channel to a resort, where they found a cache of antibiotics.

Afterward Dilan had felt a wave of joy wash over him, a feeling that was different from the adrenalin rush of doing a difficult neurosurgery. During residency, he'd been so determined to hone his surgical techniques that he'd forgotten how wonderful it felt to simply help ease another person's pain. Wasn't that why he'd wanted to become a doctor?

With that joyful feeling fresh in his mind, he returned to the States with dreams of working in Fiji a few weeks a year. He sent away for brochures and information packets. He felt more alive just thinking about it. He told Jenny about his ideas.

"That's just medical tourism," she had said, and he felt a door slam shut. Yes, he could help a few people as he'd done during his brief stay on the Yasawa Islands. But why Fiji instead of some place less exotic? Yes, it was the cool factor of flying off to the South

Pacific. He'd be just another Western doctor stepping off the plane to save the natives and relax on a nice beach. Medical tourism.

Was his desire to teach Mayegga just another expression of superiority?

The last thing Tanzania needed was another oppressor, even a well-intentioned surgeon. So many others had tried to bend these people to their wills: Arab slavers centuries ago and then, in the late 1800s, the Germans. A latecomer in Europe's race to collect colonies, Germany declared land in Tanganyika was henceforth "unowned" and herded people into labor camps. People united around a leader who believed that *maji*—a mixture of water, castor oil, and millet—would protect them. But German soldiers machine-gunned *maji* warriors row after row.

More recently, Canadian farmers had come here with their own designs. Funded by Canadian aid, they arrived on the plateau in the early 1970s with dreams of a 170,000-acre "wheat complex." They cleared massive tracts of brush and trees. Datoga people lost their most important grazing lands. "They can go to another place," the farm's research director told a British journalist.

Datoga villagers who resisted found their homes burned. Other ethnic groups were enlisted as enforcers. Datoga men were beaten and tortured with electric shocks; women were raped. Tractors plowed Datoga *bung'eda* burial tombs, which contained the remains of the Datoga's most respected elders. "When the mound is ploughed, the dead man's spirit is lost," a Datoga man told a journalist in the mid-1990s. "You don't know anymore where your father has gone. . . . We can no longer belong to this land."

For a while, the plateau was covered with golden waves of wheat, enough to make 180 million loaves of bread. But yields quickly declined. One year rats ate 80 percent of the crop; other years, great flocks of quelea birds gorged on the fields. Frustrated, the Canadians eventually sold the tracts. One day Dilan saw a tractor at the hospital. Haydom Lutheran Hospital had just bought a large parcel to start a farm.

Colonial powers and their imitators had come and gone like those brown twisters on the plateau. But the missionaries remained. Haydom was proof of their staying power. The Norwegians in 1964 handed over the hospital to the Evangelical Lutheran Church of Tanzania, but Norwegian benefactors still provided most of the hospital's funding. Foreign doctors generally held the most important positions.

Dilan thought, *If Mayegga learns brain surgery, then that would shift the paradigm.* A small shift, perhaps. Yet ripples can form waves.

But, he kept asking himself, *Is Jenny right?*

Did Mayegga really want to learn?

Was this a good thing for the hospital? Was he imposing his will on others?

He knew someone who might have answers.

CHAPTER 17

Baba Naman had taken many paths in his life, and they had usually led back to Haydom, which he loved in a way he found hard to describe. He'd grown up in Dongobesh, where his father was the first of the Iraqw people to become a Lutheran bishop. When he was young and his father was traveling, Naman grabbed his new Chinese bicycle and hit the dirt track to Haydom. Like him, the town was in its adolescence then. You could find grass huts there with alcohol and young people dancing to gramophones that spun Congolese guitar songs, perfect for a restless son of a bishop.

By the late 1960s one country after another in Africa had gained its independence. It was an exciting time, and Naman left to join the army. Starting as a supply clerk, he became a clinician and eventually a lieutenant in charge of the army's National Service health clinics. His trajectory was promising, but his mind drifted back to Haydom when his desk filled with paperwork. He thought, *I am becoming powerful, but the military can consume you. You get one promotion after another until you admire the military more than the people it serves.*

His real love was clinical medicine. So, in the early 1970s, he left the army and returned to the plateau with his new wife, Haika, a name that means "thank you" in the Chagga language. In Haydom the second Dr. Olsen taught Naman a few basic surgical procedures. And Naman would remember some of his surgery patients his entire life.

During famines patients were brought to the hospital with pieces of beans or corn in their lungs, because they had either eaten too quickly or eaten something before it was properly cooked. One day a boy of about four came in with a bean in his lung. In the operating room Naman managed to grab the bean with a bronchoscope, but then the bean fell back in. He tried a second time, and it fell again. On the third attempt, it fell into the main airway to both lungs, and he watched the boy suffocate. Devastated, he sat in the theater for half an hour, thinking about the conversation he would soon have with the parents.

But then there was Lucas, the boy whose jaw was ripped off by a hyena. Even years later, on the back patio of Mama Naman's, his eyes brightened when he thought about the boy. Lucas was about eight years old when a hyena broke through the thorns of his family's *boma*, killed his brother, and then went after him, clamping and then snapping his right arm before going for his head.

The boy arrived in Haydom with his jaw soaking in a tin cup. The second Dr. Olsen wasn't there that day, and Naman was the senior clinician in charge. He had never reattached someone's jaw but decided to try. He did his best to set the bone and wire it in place. But a few days later, the jaw turned black with rot. He removed the rotting jaw and arranged to have Lucas sent to the government hospital in Dar es Salaam.

Lucas returned a few weeks later still missing his jaw. Worse, staff in Dar es Salaam had attached two surgical gloves to his face as saliva collectors. They dangled from the sides of his mouth, dripping. Appalled, a Norwegian lab technician sent photos to journalists in Norway. "This would never happen in our country," she told Naman. The boy's story swept Norway like a spring thaw, melting hearts and exposing wallets. Soon there was enough money to fly Naman and Lucas to the southern Norwegian city of Bergen. At the hospital, Lucas was in the operating room for fourteen hours as a team of surgeons formed a new jaw from a piece of the boy's arm and put it in place.

But the new jaw began to rot again, perhaps from a lingering infection. And once again, the jaw came off. Naman escorted Lucas back to Haydom. Naman was amazed by the boy's demeanor through it all—so cheerful and intelligent! Put a new toy in his hands, and he'd figure out how it worked in an instant. And even without a jaw, you could see the smiles in his cheeks.

Six months later the Norwegian doctors tried again, and this time they succeeded. No infection; his jaw healed well. Lucas went back home to Hanang, grew up, got married, had several children, and became a carpenter. The sun had finally shone on that boy. But Naman sometimes wondered, *What if I had been able to do the surgery properly the first time? What if I had been able to save the boy with the bean lodged in his lungs?* Perhaps his fingers weren't made to operate. Healers come in many forms, not just as surgeons. Perhaps he was meant to read the shadows and light in X-rays and CT scans, find the secrets inside someone who needed help.

At Mama Naman's one night, Dilan joined Baba Naman and Mayegga on the patio. They talked about the day's surgical cases. After one of his long pauses, Dilan looked Mayegga in the eye.

"Hey, I don't want to force this on you. Is this something you really want to do?"

Mayegga looked away.

"Are you worried about something," Dilan asked.

"Yes," Mayegga finally said. "I am an AMO, not a neurosurgeon. So what will happen to me if I have a patient who has a problem? Maybe he will find a lawyer. I do not want to get into trouble."

Dilan sat with Mayegga's comments for a moment.

"I will guarantee that you will not get into trouble. If anyone has a problem, I'll deal with it."

He was taking a chance saying this. In truth, he couldn't control what happened outside the operating theater. He turned toward Baba Naman. "Dr. Naman, what do you think?"

Naman thought a moment and looked at Mayegga. "No one else can do this when Dr. Dilan leaves," he said. "So what happens to the patients then?"

"It's totally up to you," Dilan chimed in. "Should we keep doing it?"

Mayegga took a deep breath.

"OK," he said in a tentative way.

"But are you really sure?"

"Yes, yes, yes," he said, his voice rising an octave with each yes.

CHAPTER 18

_____

After three months Dilan told Mayegga, "OK, man, tomorrow I'm coming in with you but you're doing it yourself. It will be your first day as an independent neurosurgeon."

"Are you sure?" Mayegga said.

"Of course. You can do anything."

Later that night Dilan heard loud knocks on the door. It was Mayegga. He'd been drinking. His voice was loud. When Jenny tried to say something, Mayegga interrupted, "No, be silent." When Dilan tried to get a word in, Mayegga said, "I'm not done talking yet."

Dilan's heart sank. Mayegga talked for an hour about how he'd slept on cattle skins as a kid, about his work at the hospital, about other things that Dilan couldn't make out or understand. After Mayegga left, Dilan walked into town, his stomach in knots.

He found Baba Naman on the back patio of Mama Naman's restaurant. Naman looked exhausted, as if he had dozed off. But his face brightened when Dilan appeared in the door. Dilan took the seat next to him.

"I'm a little worried about Mayegga," he told Naman, and then he recounted Mayegga's visit earlier that evening. "I've given him a huge amount of information in a short time. I'm worried that the pressure is getting to him."

"Yes, he's had a hard life," Naman said. "But I don't think you need to worry. He was born to be a surgeon."

The next morning the rising sun rinsed the sky with oranges and pinks. In the theater, Dilan and Mayegga grabbed gowns and masks and went to the scrub sinks. Neither one felt like talking. Mayegga stared straight ahead as he washed his hands.

Inside Theater One a baby girl was on a bed. Her elongated head was cradled in a rolled-up towel. A nurse had covered the rest of her with a stiff green drape. Victor, the anesthesiologist, manned the hand-operated ventilator. Light filtered through the two open screen windows. Mayegga and Dilan walked in, and Dilan made sure he entered after Mayegga. Everyone gathered around the table. Mayegga looked down and said in Swahili:

"*Mwenyezi Mungo* . . . Almighty God, Father of our Lord Jesus Christ, we pray that you bless the work of our hands, lead in this operation, bless our patient, that she might be able to benefit from recovery after this surgery. We ask this through our Lord Jesus Christ, your son. Amen."

Dilan stepped back from the table, out of the first zone. He stretched his hands out as if handing him something. *It's all yours.*

Mayegga's eyes widened.

"Are you sure?"

Dilan nodded, yes.

Mayegga turned to the girl, and with his right hand, reached for a No. 10 scalpel. Holding it like a pencil, he made a small U-shaped incision above the child's forehead as Dilan had taught. Mayegga looked up.

"Perfect," Dilan said.

Mayegga's left hand held a white sponge to capture the blood from the incision. He pulled off a flap of skin and tissue to expose the bone. He picked up the Hudson Brace, centered it in the incision, and turned the crank. It squeaked with every revolution.

"You can go a little faster," Dilan said.

The rhythmic squeaks from the drill increased.

"But don't push in too hard. You don't want to plunge it into the middle of the brain." *Let him know that this is serious. A surgeon who feels no fear is dangerous.*

Mayegga felt the bit go through the harder surface of the skull, then the softer part. He felt the bit catch and eased off the pressure. Through the bone. Another quarter turn. Done.

Now Mayegga could see the lining of the brain through the hole. He usually didn't sweat in the theater, but pearls formed now on his forehead. He asked a nurse to wipe them away.

He cauterized some tissue. He picked up the IV tube and inserted it into the child's brain. Fluid flowed out the other end.

"Way to go," Dilan said.

By now, eight other nurses and clinical officers had entered the room. Dilan took another step back as the Tanzanians moved into the inner zone. *Mayegga's success will be their success*, Dilan thought. He peered over their shoulders to make sure everything was OK.

Mayegga took the tube and with a long set of forceps worked it underneath the skin of the child's neck, down through the chest, and into the child's belly.

Dilan stepped back from the table altogether; then he paced around the edge of the room; then he said he'd once seen a surgeon do a similar operation and get something tangled inside the patient's brain. That patient had died. *He should know this is a big deal, that he's doing something that experienced surgeons sometimes mess up.* Two hours passed. Mayegga was about to close.

"Dr. Mayegga, what do you think? Are you happy?"

"Yes, yes, sure," Mayegga replied, eyes still locked on his patient.

Dilan strode to the door. He yanked off his mask, ripped off his gloves and gown, and tossed everything into a corner. He smacked his hands together, and the clap echoed across the room. The nurses and clinicians started clapping; the women ululated. *Yi! Yi! Yi!*

Dilan opened the double door. In a voice he knew would carry down the halls, he shouted, "Now you've got a neurosurgeon!"

CHAPTER 19

The dry season ended slowly and in a teasing way, first with the appearance of green leaves on the acacias, even though no rain had come and without any promise that it would. The leaves grew on faith, and people acted on faith as well; farmers and schoolchildren turned the hard red earth with their picks. Gray clouds moved in, left behind a few encouraging drops, then flew away.

And then the rains returned and settled in, and suddenly everything around Haydom was wet. The fissures in the road filled with water; water coursed down the hill behind the hospital. The twisters on the plateau vanished. In the fields, the farmers and the schoolchildren seeded the moist soil with sunflowers and maize. The soil changed from bright red to brownish red, the color of a healing scab.

When it rained, patients and their families sought shelter underneath a roof overhang by Radiology. They sat on long benches and took off their sandals and shoes. They crossed their arms and wrapped themselves tightly in *shuka* blankets until the storms passed. Then the sun broke through, and everything glistened. Around the wards, purple jacaranda blossoms filled the trees. Red bougainvillea bushes bloomed around the cottages for the visiting doctors. To Dilan, this luxuriant air and vegetation reminded him of the jungles around Kandy. He felt a change in himself; he'd arrived in Haydom wrung dry. Now he sensed something new, a sense of possibility, a chance that his life someday could be full, even overflowing.

·   ·   ·

It had taken time to mend, for it all to clot. But as the months passed, he found this place more energizing and healing than he ever expected. Every piece of broken equipment was an opportunity to try something new.

When the original tree saw broke, he found orthopedic wire and twisted them together to make a new one.

When he couldn't find pieces of collagen mesh, he took sutures, cut off the needle parts, and stuffed the tangles on patients' brain tissues.

When suction devices didn't work, he used syringes. He used duct tape to hold appliances together. He had mechanics in the garage fashion special metal plates for patients with cervical fractures. Anything was possible. You just had to think outside that closed box.

As their time in Haydom grew shorter, he and Jenny sometimes found themselves on the road to Haydom town at night, though Dilan increasingly went alone. Once full of dust, the road now was full of puddles. He'd come to realize how much he loved that everything around Haydom was unpaved. In America, pavement was one of its defining features. But on the way to Mama Naman's, you felt the ruts and smooth parts, heard the crunch of your feet, the slopping noise when you stepped in a puddle. You were connected. He spent hours at Mama Naman's restaurant, joining others as they crowded into the bar to hear the news on Baba Naman's television. Now and then one of the channels broadcast an old speech by Julius Nyerere, *mwalimu*, "teacher," the country's beloved first president. Sometimes, Mayegga joined Dilan on the back patio, finding a seat that gave him a view of the horizon.

During those nights Dilan thought about the friends he'd made here, and the thought of leaving filled him with sadness. He would leave them behind, and increasingly, he knew he would leave his relationship with Jenny behind as well.

For a time, he thought they would be married. But in the end, they were too much alike, two strings playing the same note, competing with one another instead of harmonizing. She left Haydom two months before him, done with her elective.

He was alone. Again. And that somehow was OK.

Just before he left Haydom, he told Mayegga, "Now you have to start teaching someone else. Start with radiology, and pick a clinical officer, or an AMO, and teach them how to do CT scans. Do it the same way I taught you."

Soon he would be nine thousand miles away from Haydom, directing a neurotrauma center in Oregon. He would be a junior attending physician, assistant professor, teaching residents what he'd been taught a few years before. Back on his career track, back on something paved.

From Haydom, he went to Zanzibar to collect his thoughts, or rather, let them go for a few more weeks. In the cobalt waters, he washed away what was left of Haydom's reddish earth. He dove into the Indian Ocean with an oxygen tank on his back and swam through seawater that was impossibly blue.

PART 2

Do One

The value of experience is not in seeing much, but in seeing wisely.

—WILLIAM OSLER, Canadian physician and cofounder of Johns Hopkins Hospital

In 1984 a famine in Ethiopia spawned a new movement: music for the poor. Moved by television footage of starving refugees, super-groups formed to sing "Do They Know It's Christmas" and "We Are the World." The songs sold by the millions. In 1985 two billion people watched the Live Aid concerts. Bob Geldof, one of the organizers, said later that these campaigns made "compassion hip."

All of this happened amid a new economic force that would shape how legions of people in wealthy countries helped the poor—a decline in international airfares.

Per mile, fares dropped to a third of what they were in the 1960s, triggering an explosion in global tourism. In 1950 tourists took about twenty-five million international trips; sixty years later, visitors went on nearly one billion. Those who grew up listening to "We Are the World" could now find convenient ways to visit the world's poor, often in the form of short-term missions.

Many of these missions were organized by churches, which used group trips as vehicles to spread the gospel and strengthen the bonds of its members. In 1989 about 125,000 American Christians went on short-term missions. By 2005 the number exceeded 1.6 million. All told, these traveling volunteers spent an estimated $2.4 billion. And as more contrails appeared over Africa and South America, the notion of what it meant to be a missionary began to change.

For centuries, missionaries left their countries behind for years or for the rest of their lives. But with cheaper airfares, people suddenly could do missions on their vacations and school breaks. By the mid-2000s, nearly one-third of all American teens had done religious service missions. In North America, short-term missions became the biggest competitors to summer camps. Exotic places were popular destinations. The Bahamas received one short-term missionary for every fifteen residents. Over time, the purpose of many missions shifted away from sacrifice toward self-enrichment. "Let's be honest," said David Livermore, executive director of the Global Learning Center at Grand Rapids Theological Seminary. "Along with the seemingly more noble reasons for going on a short-term mission trip, many of us love the adventure of it all."

Doctors, nurses, and medical students were an important subset of this larger short-term mission trend. Some went with church groups, but many also went on trips sponsored by universities and teaching hospitals, as Jenny had. In 1984 only one of seventeen graduating American medical students did overseas medical training. By the late 2000s the number was one in three.

Many cited these trips as a way to reconnect with the reasons they went into medicine—to help those truly in need. They came back with stories about horrible working conditions and a new appreciation of what they had at home. They talked about the freedom of working in places without the insurance and liability headaches of the Western medical industry.

With so much demand, an industry grew up to facilitate these medical trips, sometimes pitching them with sweeteners: "This trip includes a day of rest at the beach! You are just a short plane ride away from some of the most famous World Heritage Sites," one medical NGO said about its excursion to Nicaragua. Another touted its Kenya "Out of Africa experience!" and how Maasai warriors would greet you "with a simple 'Jambo' or 'hello.'" All told, doctors and students went on about six thousand short-term missions a year, spending at least $250 million. In a generation, medical missions had become hip.

A year after Dilan's departure from Haydom, Carin Hoek stepped out of Radiology and moved toward the light. Dark rooms made her sleepy, and the morning meeting had left her eyelids heavy, though in a pleasant way. The soft voices of the Tanzanian clinicians sounded like distant chants, and the X-rays on the light board came and went like moon phases.

Carin's green clogs squeaked on the hallway's red cement as she made her way to the open door outside. She passed benches where patients in purple and red blankets slept like sideways question marks. When she stepped into the courtyard, the sunlight hit her retinas with such force that everything seemed overbright. Her pupils raced to adjust, hurting a little, generating tears, and she thought, *Isn't it delightful to feel the sun's sudden embrace?*

She joined Anderson Sakweli, a Tanzanian clinician with a wide face and eyes that moved back and forth like a school of fish. She had heard that Sakweli could be dismissive, especially with women. But Carin looked at his broad face and thought, *I'll win him over.* She would do it first by calling him *daktari*, the Swahili word for doctor, even though he was an assistant medical officer. A few foreign doctors had corrected her: "Oh, Sakweli, he's not a real doctor, by the way." But she pretended not to hear them. He did *daktari* work, so she would call him *daktari*. Even better, she would call him *mwalimu*, "teacher."

"*Mwalimu*, may I follow you?"

"Of course," he said. "It will be a pleasure."

The more she caught his moving eyes, the more compassion and kindness she saw in them. Curt with foreigners? Easy to see why. So many visitors came and went. She wasn't one of them. She had a contract to work in Haydom for at least two years. "Maybe I'll stay longer," she told herself. "Maybe forever." This place, its light and colors and movement—it was so different from the Netherlands. But it already felt like home.

Carin Hoek was Haydom Lutheran Hospital's new pediatrician, here to run the Lena children's ward. It was her first day of rounds. A big day for her, and for the ward. Volunteer doctors had come for a month here and there, but until today, the Lena Ward had never had a full-time pediatrician. Sakweli had been left to do what he could. As she and Sakweli crossed the compound, she walked a half step behind as a sign of respect. A red dirt path cut through a courtyard of dry grass. The busy surgical ward was on their left; the tuberculosis ward was a few steps farther. People milled outside both buildings. In the courtyard, women spread *kangas* on the dry grass; men with purple *shukas* over their shoulders leaned on their herding staffs. They all stared at her as she walked toward them, and she smiled back. She smiled often, and when she did, it sent creases upward and out from her blue eyes. It was a smile enhanced by her height: five-foot-ten with long arms and legs sculpted from rowing around The Hague. Her posture was arrow straight. She had short, fine blonde hair that glowed when struck by a sunbeam. It combed easily and scattered just as easily when hit by gusts. Her voice was airy and full of movement, formal one minute, a burst of words another. She finished sentences with light laughs, which put others, as well as herself, at ease.

The glass doors to Lena Ward were locked, so Sakweli banged on the window. The head janitor appeared and clicked open the door, looking at Sakweli first and then the floor. The door opened into a spacious playroom. Its walls were covered with hand-painted cartoons of lions, zebras, and monkeys. The room was empty. Where were all the children? At any given time, the ward was supposed to house 150 or more.

She set the question aside as she spotted a framed photograph just above another set of double doors. It was a young Norwegian girl named Lena Slogedal Paulsen. She had blonde hair that curled around her face in a heart shape and a heart-shaped locket around her neck. Carin had heard her story the day before.

Lena was ten years old in 2000, walking on a lake path in southern Norway with an eight-year-old friend, when two men asked if they wanted to see some kittens. The men took them behind some bushes, raped the girls, and then stabbed them to death. The crimes and trials of the young men shocked the entire country. Later, Lena's grieving mother read a newspaper story about Haydom's crowded children's wards and discovered a cause: little Lena had talked about how she would help the poor when she grew up. Lena's mother launched a campaign that raised $350,000 to build a new children's ward in Haydom. Lena kept her promise.

Carin made a mental note to say a prayer for the family. And one for herself. She could easily lose herself in the horror of Lena's death, and that wouldn't help any of the children she was about to see.

They opened the doors to the ward, and suddenly the quiet of the playroom merged with a wave of noise: shrieking babies, nurses calling to each other, the slurp of a mop moving across the hallway floor. The scents hit her next: sweat, urine, diarrhea, and soapy water. Above the doors were signs with handwritten black letters: No 1. Malnutrition, No 2. Malnutrition, No. 3. Malaria. For a moment she struggled to take it all in.

The nursing station was on the right. She breathed a bit easier. In hospitals everywhere, nursing stations were sanctuaries. Away from the patients, you could chat about relationships, food, and hospital gossip, catch your breath. Nurses in white uniforms circled around a long wooden table in the center of the room. Angela, the head nurse, leaned against the table, her head buried in a ledger. She didn't look up.

"*Shikamoo*, Nursi Angela," Carin said, a polite way of greeting people in Tanzania that means, "May I kiss your feet?" Tanzanians typically replied, "*Marahaba* (I'm delighted)," a way of accepting the greeting. Angela kept her eyes fixed on the ledger.

Angela was an elegant woman with smooth brown skin and eyebrows that arched like two triangles. Carin had met her the day before, and she had been chilly then, too. No, she looked tired, with a face that seemed to say, "Not another one." Carin thought, *Ah, she's like Sakweli. Every new visitor means more questions, more work. Well, I'll show her that I'm different.*

Sakweli finished his conversation with Angela, and without signaling to Carin, started his rounds. She followed him to a room at the far end of the ward. As Sakweli stood near the door, Angela ordered the children back to their beds, then handed him a clipboard.

"Is the child improving?" he asked, flipping through medication forms and a sheet with the child's vitals.

"Yes," the nurse answered. "The child is improving."

Sakweli moved to another child, looked at the chart.

"Is the child improving?"

"Yes, the child is improving."

To Carin's eyes, some of the children looked as if they wouldn't last the night; rail thin, they had the faraway gazes of prison inmates. A few children did indeed look well, but Sakweli made no move to discharge them. Odd. The ward was full; shouldn't they discharge these healthy children to make more room?

A voice in her mind said, "Wait, Ca. Just wait."

OK, I'll wait. She would keep her hands behind her back, ask Sakweli basic questions: What steps do you take to diagnose a patient with malaria? How do you decide whether a patient has TB? Happy questions, ones that told Sakweli "I'm here to learn, not lecture you about how I did things in the Netherlands."

In the next room the children had bloated bellies and terrible edemas. "If you are wondering whether this is a kidney edema or malnutrition, look at their expressions," Sakweli said. "If their eyes show despair, it is malnutrition, kwashiorkor."

Carin stared at a baby girl with big brown eyes, a swollen belly, and patches of hair; her brows were shaped in two pleading squiggles. Sakweli moved to another room with more starving children. Sometimes Sakweli spoke so softly that she could barely hear him. Her legs began to ache; her muscles grew stiff when she observed others; and her mind mimicked her hair in the wind, scattering even as she tried to move it back in place. *Yes, the cottage needs work; I need to mend the holes in the mosquito net. What about Emma? She's leaving soon. What do you give someone who leaves Haydom?* When the tasks grew too numerous to remember, she took out a pen and scribbled notes on her arm. Soon her arm was full of temporary tattoos.

"Aaaieeee!" A child's scream brought her back. They rushed to an open door. Carin smelled decay and soap. Two nurses were next to a galvanized tub that contained a girl who looked to be about eight years old. She had the same swooping eyebrows as Angela's. The girl's eyes were full of tears. She had bandages around her torso, shoulder, and left arm. Her legs were missing from her knees down; the stumps were wrapped in gauze.

"*Pole sana, basi, pole sana* (sorry, all right then, sorry)," the nurses said as they unwrapped another bandage. The girl's scream rose like a wave, then broke into a foam of sobs and shallow breaths. Her exposed flesh was black and pink. A few feet away, her brother watched with wide eyes. His back was charred from his buttocks to his neck. He was next.

"Oh, what happened?" Carin asked.

"Burns," Angela said. A pot of boiling oil fell on them. The girl lost her legs, but they were both on a list to get skin grafts. A plastic surgeon from California sometimes visited and did grafts. And the AMO named Mayegga also knew how to do them.

"Angela, this suffering breaks my heart. Do these children get any pain medication?"

"Oh, yes, we give them acetaminophen."

Carin smiled back, but this one was forced. Acetaminophen? Tylenol? That's for fevers and headaches. In the Netherlands, they put patients under when dressing severe burns. She moved her hands from behind her back to the front. Painkillers, where are the painkillers?

Wait, Ca, wait. Put it on the list.

Still shaken, Carin followed Sakweli and Angela to neonatology, which doubled as the orphanage. By the wall, a high table contained a row of babies. A few of their faces had bluish-gray tints. *They're hypoxic!*

Another table of babies was across the room, the orphans. Some had rolled onto each other's blankets. They looked healthy. Trying to be positive, Carin said to an older nurse named Mama Kidogo, "The orphans look very happy."

"Their tears run inside," Mama Kidogo replied.

Carin looked at the premature babies struggling for oxygen, and then back at the orphans who had equally uncertain futures. Like divorcing parents, the arguments in her mind grew louder. *Make changes*, she thought. *Immediately*. Then the voice again, that damn voice. "Wait, Ca, wait. For at least six months." But how could she wait? Even for a minute? Don't these children deserve the best care possible? Now?

"Please excuse me," she said. When her mind overflowed like this in the Netherlands, she fled to the beach, especially if the weather was gray and windy. Then the beach would be empty and she could face the wind and sing and scream into it, and because the ripping wind drowned everything but her own voice, it was just her and her thoughts. She could sort through the ones that mattered. Was there a place like this in Haydom?

She left through the double doors, passing Lena's photograph. She marched back to her cottage, thinking about the children and then the Flying Medical Service plane she'd arrived in the day before. *Yes, the airstrip.*

She exchanged her clogs for running shoes and followed the dirt driveway to the hospital gates. *Was it right to stand by and let a child suffer? I could have done something.* Her mentor's voice again: "No, dear, they managed for decades without you. Aren't you really trying to comfort yourself?"

When she reached the airstrip, she pulled out a pink moleskin notebook and crouched on one knee. She used her knee as a desk and jotted notes about procedures and protocols she wanted to change. In a few moments, she filled several pages with scribbles and arrows and underlined words. Then she walked briskly back to her cottage, tore the pages from the notebook, and stuffed them in a wooden nightstand. She sealed the drawer with duct tape, then stood straight, took a deep breath, and burst into laughter.

Her mentor had been right all along.

CHAPTER 21

Everything had changed in a flash, as if the wind had caught some long-smoldering ember.

Two months before, Carin was running an entire surgical wing at Juliana Children's Hospital in The Hague. Light and airy and with lots of finished wood, that hospital was near the ocean, close enough to feel the churn of the dark green waters. Carin had found she liked the night shift the best there. At night the hospital's pulse slowed, and you had more time to check on slumbering children or softly tell a new mother, "Your baby is beautiful, everything is OK." Not all nights were quiet, of course. A sudden squall of patients might fill the emergency room. But even then the night rhythm was different, and so was she, lost in the flow of tasks and goals, calm and efficient, as if rowing hard in still water. Later, when it was quiet again, she walked through the hallways feeling like a captain on a great ship, surrounded by dark seas and moving with great momentum toward daybreak.

She was twenty-nine years old, unusually young to have such responsibility so soon out of residency, the start of a promising career. She loved the hospital and her colleagues there, but she'd found herself asking, *Am I really needed here?* The Netherlands had many good pediatricians. The more she thought about the future, the darker it felt. *OK, when do I feel the most light?*

The answer came in an instant—Wednesday nights. On Wednesdays, she took a yellow train from The Hague to the center of Amsterdam, then, usually late, she rushed to a course in tropical medicine. Here she learned the medical names for starvation— kwashiorkor and marasmus. She learned how Rift Valley fever enslaved its victims and left them vomiting blood. Roundworms blocked the lymphatic system, triggering elephantiasis, which caused people's arms, legs, and genitals to quadruple in size. Small black flies caused river blindness; dengue fever made legs and arms feel as if they'd been whacked by tire irons. Even diarrhea was fascinating: in the Netherlands, flu viruses, improperly handled food, and allergies were your likely suspects. But in great swaths of Africa, South America, and Asia, any number of intestinal dragons could invade your gut.

One rainy weekend she went to a tropical medicine conference, arriving late as usual. She tossed her umbrella near a door and slipped into the auditorium. She spotted friends from Juliana and squeezed into a seat next to them. In between a presentation, the director of Tweega Medica Foundation took the stage: a hospital in a remote area in Tanzania needed a doctor for two years. Would anyone in the audience be interested?

Carin sat with the idea for a moment. *A doctor in Africa.* Then a vision formed in her mind, diffuse but inevitable, like sunlight just before it breaks over the horizon. She raised her hand. "Cut it out, Ca, what are you doing?" a friend next to her said. But she kept her hand up, and then raised it higher.

Soon, she had sold or given away most of her things and stuffed an enormous red Samsonite suitcase with books, a laptop, donated medical equipment, sunscreen, duct tape, clothes for a year, camping gear, antibiotics, journals, earrings, a Bible, a poetry book, a camera, makeup, and scissors to cut her own hair. She had nothing against medical students who went on short-term missions; she had long thought that students and colleagues who went on these trips returned with brighter looks on their faces. But in her mind, this wasn't a trip. It was a move.

A few friends tried to discourage her; they set her up on blind dates, hoping she would fall in love and stay. They said, "Ca, you're going to end up an old maid. You're going to the bush; you'll never meet a man you'll want to marry." But she had made up her mind. When she arrived in Africa and listed her occupation on various immigration forms, she wrote, "Missionary Doctor."

· · ·

Before Haydom, she spent a month in Malawi with one of the world's most respected missionary doctors, Elizabeth Molyneux. Professor Molyneux had a round face, shiny skin, and gray hair that she parted in the middle. She was from Great Britain and had moved to Malawi in 1974 with her husband, a noted malaria researcher. Her serene but firm look reminded Carin of Mother Superior in *The Sound of Music*. In her research, Molyneux had discovered that clinicians in Malawi often failed to diagnose children with leukemia because its symptoms were so similar to malaria. Worse, children with cancer were often brought to hospitals and clinics too late to be treated. And not just in Malawi. Across the world, eight of ten children with cancer received substandard care or no care at all.

Professor Molyneux also discovered that you could increase cancer survival rates if you simplified treatment protocols—broke them into parts and mastered each process. Clarity and simplicity led to quality, and not just when it came to cancer. The creation of an accident and emergency unit with streamlined triage procedures cut the number of child deaths by nearly 20 percent. Molyneux had everyone sit in a circle during morning meetings, local and foreign doctors alike, and then went over cases in amazing depth; doctors were expected to find out what foods were cooked in a child's home, whether the family used wood or gas, when children went to bed. You could make 80 percent of your diagnoses simply by asking questions and listening to patients and their families. This was important in low-income countries where lab tests were unavailable or of questionable quality. You used what you had, and what you often had were the people in front of you. Carin took so many notes that she had to buy extra notebooks.

On her last day, she found Molyneux in her office. "You operate such a wonderful department here," she told the professor. "Would it be possible for me to have a copy of your protocols?"

Molyneux leaned forward and pressed her hands together. "Dr. Hoek, I'm not going to give you any of my protocols." Carin felt two feet shorter.

"I started out just like you. On my own. Out in the bush. The worst thing you could do is to bring a set of protocols and start implementing them. The most important thing to do is make friends, real friends. Find out what makes them happy, and what keeps them awake at night. And in the hospital, you might be shocked by what you see. But, you must wait. Make a list. When you feel the urge to change something, write down your ideas. Then put the list into a drawer and lock it. Wait six months before opening it. If your ideas still make sense after this time, then make those changes. By then, you will have the support of your staff." With that, the professor wished her well.

Later that night, Carin thought, *What if the professor's protocols saved someone's life?* She borrowed a friend's bicycle and rode to the hospital. With a camera and a flashlight, she went from room to room, feeling like a spy. She took snapshots of the protocols on the walls, thirty-seven lists in all. When she was done, she still had to pass the professor's office. The door was closed. She walked by on light feet, whispering, "Professor, I will put these protocols to good use. I promise."

Then she whispered to herself, "Ca, you will wait and wait."

Weeks after her arrival in Haydom, Carin glanced at the drawer with the duct-tape seal and mouthed a silent thank-you.

Had she blurted out her ideas during her first days, she would have looked arrogant and naïve—another *mzungu* telling Sakweli and Angela how to run things. You had to spend time in the nursing station to see Angela prop herself in a chair after an exhausting shift—how Angela and the other nurses earned the dark circles under their eyes by spending hours ventilating babies who often died anyway; you had to help the nurses intubate one child after another, then join them for a break in the nursing station, before they opened up about their families or revealed how some had trained in Norway, thanks to the hospital's sponsorship, how they could have left Haydom for better-paying jobs but stayed because they felt responsible for their people.

Professor Molyneux's advice to wait and wait also had bought Carin time to discover the Lena Ward's little mysteries. Why was the playroom so empty? Because healthy Tanzanian children play outside. Why didn't Sakweli discharge the healthy children that morning? Because their parents hadn't paid their bills. The malnourished children? They truly were improving.

The professor's admonition "to wait and wait" also gave her a chance to study the visiting doctors and students, who both inspired and troubled her.

CHAPTER 22

In a few weeks, Carin's Swahili became more fluent. Things that once seemed abnormal were completely normal: a man lugging three dead chickens past your table at the Two Sisters just after you ordered chicken *kuku*; a cattle herd roaming through the hospital compound to keep the grass down; paying a patient's bills—once you did that for one child you had to do it for others. As her new Haydom-shaped neural pathways grew stronger, she saw the visiting doctors and students in a different way.

Many were adventurous people with big hearts. Their open faces and clear eyes showed how much they wanted to help. Time and again, she heard them say:

"I came here to give something back."

Inevitably, they added, "But I think I gained more out of this than they did."

But some cloaked positive statements with veils of superiority:

"The people are so happy here, even though they are so poor."

"They do so much here with so little. It shows us how much we have at home."

And others just rolled their eyes.

"They just don't care."

"They value life differently here."

She began to think about the term *expat*. It had an air of Western privilege to it. Why were visiting workers in Africa called expats, while in Europe and North America they were called migrants and immigrants? Over and over in the Netherlands, she'd heard native Dutch people complain about its growing population of immigrants, or *gastarbeider*, Dutch for "guest workers." No one ever called them expatriates. So, half-teasing, she started describing herself as a guest worker. Doing this somehow made things feel more balanced.

Carin found that some doctors didn't plant deep roots in Haydom even when they stayed for long periods. Case in point was Emma, a colleague from the Netherlands. She was in Haydom for a year to work in Lena Ward and do a clubfoot treatment project. Emma had cured a large number of children by doing a series of casts to force their feet back into the proper positions. The world was full of famous people who had once had clubfoot: Olympic figure skater Kristi Yamaguchi, American soccer star Mia Hamm. But in sub-Saharan Africa, parents often lacked access to clinics that did such casts. As a result, children grew up as invalids, limping perhaps with the help of a stick. Emma had tried to teach the Tanzanian staff how to make the casts, but had given up. "They just don't do it right," she told Carin one day. It was much easier to do the job herself. Then with an urgency that caught Carin off guard, she added, "You must promise me that you'll keep doing this when I'm gone."

Emma was as devoted a doctor as Carin had ever seen, but the suffering in the wards had filled Emma with despair. Her despair burned like a wildfire at times, consuming everything in its path, including the sensitivities of the Tanzanian staff. She ordered them around and sighed in exasperation when they didn't meet her expectations. When they felt she went too far, they woke her up in the night about an emergency. She rushed to the ward but found no emergency at all; it was payback. Now she was exhausted. She was glad to go, and she knew the Tanzanians were glad to see her leave. Her eyes filled with tears as she told Carin, "Don't give them too much. They'll swallow you."

Not long after Emma left Haydom, Carin received a text from the clinician Emmanuel Mayegga: an eight-year-old boy was on the way, airway obstruction, emergency. Carin rushed to the Lena Ward's ICU and collected nasogastric tubes, an oxygen tank, mask and balloon, IV needles, saline, a pulse oximeter, and adrenaline.

A Land Cruiser ambulance raced through the hospital gates. The driver had gone full tilt for three hours across sixty kilometers of bush. The boy arrived with his parents, who looked as if lost in another country. Their son's face was gray.

Quickly, Carin pieced together what happened: After a bout of diarrhea, the boy was dehydrated and listless. To boost his energy, his parents gave him sugar powder, which probably contained cornstarch. But he accidentally inhaled it, and the powder turned to glue when it mixed with the moisture in his lungs. It triggered a bronchial spasm. Now, he could inhale, but the air didn't come out, which meant he was suffocating; he writhed on the bed like a fish on a boat deck.

"Get me an IV," she told Mayegga. "And administer epinephrine and salbutamol."

A mnemonic trick flashed through her mind: O2: ABC—Oxygen: Airway, Breathing, Circulation.

She pinned the boy to the bed and put her ear to his mouth. Nothing. She placed a stethoscope on his chest. A sound: a tight wheezing noise, deep in the lungs, similar to a lethal asthma attack.

O2: ABC. We're stuck at B.

The boy's eyes were wet with panic. She tried to ventilate him with an oxygen bag. No air went in. His eyes turned upward, and he began to shake.

"Angela, give him a sedative. We need to stop the convulsions."

Quick injection. The boy stopped moving his arms and legs, then stopped breathing.

I'm losing him.

Asthma? Anoxia? Lack of oxygen to the brain. A memory, a conversation with a Dutch pediatric intensive-care doctor, a well-built guy, hearty laugh. He'd told her about a child with a severe asthma attack. He tried everything he could to get oxygen into the child's lungs, but nothing worked. In desperation, he placed his hands on the boy's thorax and pumped hard—a crazy thing to do, but it did the trick.

Carin wasn't sure whether the story was true. The doctor was known to embellish. But every conversation about a patient is an opportunity to learn. She looked at the boy on the table. *I can't just stand here and do nothing as he dies.* She told Angela to put an oxygen mask over the boy's mouth. Emmanuel Mayegga stood nearby.

"Get ready," she told Angela. She placed her hand on the boy's thorax. With all her might, she pushed down.

"Expiration!" she shouted.

"Inspiration!" Carin shouted as Angela squeezed the oxygen bag. She meant to say *ventilation*, but *inspiration* was her Dutch-to-English translation.

Carin pushed down again. "Expiration!"

"Inspiration!" Angela squeezed again.

Carin looked at the pulse oximeter. It measured oxygen levels. One hundred was normal. Seventy and below meant you were dying. It said thirty.

"Expiration!"

"Inspiration!"

On her third try, the number ticked up. Ten minutes passed, then twenty. *Keep going. Never give up hope.* She glanced at Mayegga, whose eyes were fixed on the pulse oximeter. It was above fifty.

"Expiration!"

"Inspiration!"

Suddenly the boy coughed. Thick plugs of mucus and sugar popped out. The color poured back into his face.

Mayegga stood back and looked amused.

"That is something new," he said.

"No credit to me. God helped him through," Carin answered with a smile.

Later she thought about how close that boy had come to death. Only a stray memory deep in her brain had saved him, a single conversation about a patient. Maybe it was Providence that she found that memory. Or maybe it was just luck. She was certain about one thing. Hope was why she was here to help nurses like Angela; hope was why she kept thumping on the boy's chest; hope was why he was kicking a soccer ball now under the jacaranda trees outside the ward. Emma had warned, "Don't give them too much."

But Carin told herself, *I will give every ounce I possibly can.*

CHAPTER 23

On a dark porch in Portland, Oregon, Dilan struck a match: friction, ignition, a sound like a newspaper tear, and a flame. He brought the flame closer to his face and then to the tip of a cigarette, a Camel. He inhaled and filled his lungs. Bitter smoke, so different from the wood smoke that set his mind ablaze in Africa; these particles did nothing but reinforce his funk. *I'm so homesick.*

Portland was a city of coffee, Gore-Tex, and mist. He'd rented a house in a gentrified neighborhood a short drive from Oregon Health and Science University. With Jenny out of his life, he was alone this evening, though not really free. He was on call. Being on call meant you couldn't go out of town, commit to a movie—commit to much of anything other than your cell phone, which buzzed soon enough.

It was the chief resident in the OR. Paramedics had wheeled in a young woman.

"Bad car accident," the resident said. "Subdural hemorrhage, blown pupil, acutely herniated, she's intubated."

"OK, pack her up. I'll meet you in the OR." Relief. Something to move his mind from the past to now.

He changed into his scrubs, locked up, and climbed into an old gray Saab with a drooping headliner. He'd tried to tack up the headliner with a medical staple gun but only made it look worse. He gunned the engine, put the car in gear, and sped toward a cluster of buildings on a hill. It was late evening, and the sodium-vapor street lamps cast light the color of liquid nicotine.

This would be one of his first trauma cases in Oregon. Time to set the bar, get the nurses used to his pace, get everyone battle ready, especially the medical students and residents. If any were the least bit unkempt, he would bark at them like a drill sergeant. "You're a doctor now, button that coat. Act like a doctor." No excuses for forgetting a minor vital sign; details matter when your margin of error is zero.

Ahead on the hill, he spotted the glowing glass windows of OHSU. A new Swiss-made aerial tram connected the hospital with a doctors' office building below the hill. Traffic was light, and he was inside the ER within ten minutes, locked and loaded, no time for hellos.

"Is the patient in?" he asked the nurse outside the trauma bay.

She stiffened at his tone. "Just rolled into the OR."

The patient was on a gurney. Nurses and residents fluttered about like moths around a bulb.

"Everyone, stop what you're doing! Now!"

The residents squared their shoulders; the nurses braced.

It could take an hour and a half to prep a patient for brain surgery. This woman had forty minutes, max. The blown pupil was the clue. It meant that tissues had herniated and were pressing on the brain stem. *Time is brain.*

"Look, we have a chance to save a life. What we do in the next few minutes will determine whether she lives or dies."

He faced the scrub nurse.

"No time for a full tray. I need five things now: suction, scalpel, Bovie, Raney clips, knife. Leave everything else." Ten minutes of brain saved.

He turned to the anesthesiologist.

"Put in your lines as we operate." Ten more minutes saved.

To the junior resident: "Shave the head and pour Betadine all over it. That's all the prep you're gonna do." Four minutes saved.

To another resident pinning the woman's head in a Mayfield clamp: "Forget the pins." They would use a rolled-up towel, as he'd done in Haydom. Two minutes saved.

I'll make up the rest on my own.

He grabbed a scalpel, cut quickly. Now the pneumatic drill. Whirring noise, bone flecks. Bone flap off. Inside her skull, hunting for the hemorrhage. *There it is.* Bovie knife, the sizzle of cauterized tissue. Sealed, fixed, now close and check the clock.

Thirty minutes.

He stepped away from the table.

"Hey, I know I was pushing you. But today we gave this young woman a chance. Well done, everyone. Well done."

He walked out, double-barrel eyes, eyes like the surgeon in the poster he put on his wall when he was a teen. Blood coursed through his veins. This was the joy of surgery, why he'd trained so long. And now the cases were coming at him like gunfire.

Another night on call, another night pacing on the porch thinking about Haydom. His phone buzzed, thank heaven. The chief resident: "Dilan, you won't believe this. We've got a guy with an arrow through his orbit."

"What?"

"Yeah, a crossbow bolt. Just missed the man's left eye, but it went through the frontal cortex."

"Is he dead?"

By dead, he meant, was he too far gone for surgery? Get the punch line up-front.

"No, he's alert and talking, knows where he is and what's going on. He can even see out of that left eye."

"On my way."

By the time he arrived the resident had done a CT scan and an angiogram. Dilan studied the images. The arrowhead had gone through the superior and posterior aspect of the orbit and into the inferior left frontal lobe, across the midline, to the right frontal lobe. The tip was lodged in the Sylvian fissure. *Good thing it missed the anterior cerebral artery*, he thought. *Lucky dude.* Had that bolt gone in a millimeter to the right, he would be in the morgue. He might still end up there because of that arrowhead.

Look at that artery. The notch in the arrowhead had slipped under the vessel like a fish hook. Yank out the arrow and the artery would come with it. The guy would die on the table.

He'd heard about people getting hit with arrows in Haydom. One time Baba Naman had a patient come in with an arrow sticking out of his head. Somehow Naman arranged to fly him to Dar es Salaam, where a surgeon successfully pulled it out. But in Portland?

He studied the patient's CT, memorized the angles, then scrubbed in. He thought about what could go wrong. Odds are he would rupture that artery. Then he would have to do an emergency craniotomy. There would be massive bleeding. He was fast, but probably not fast enough to stop such a dam burst. The OR team was ready with the suckers. They brought in liters of extra blood. He slipped on a thin surgical glove instead of the thicker orthopedic ones he normally used—he needed more tactile control.

He held the shaft with his fingertip, then pushed it in deeper to unhook the artery. He pictured the artery in his mind and the anatomy around it. *Get the angles right, or this guy's toast.* He pressed sideways on the shaft to make the exit angle different from the entry angle. *Gotta clear that artery.* He pulled it out a few millimeters. No tension tugging on the shaft. *Keep going.* A few more millimeters. *OK, go for it.*

He slid the arrow out like a straw from a cup.

Eye saved, brain saved, life saved.

How about that? he said to himself as he walked out of the OR. *I just pulled an arrow out of a dude's head.* He wouldn't have to crack open the guy's skull after all. He thought of George Patton, who once said, "Compared to war all other forms of human endeavor shrink to insignificance. God, I do love it so!" Yeah, but Patton never did brain surgery.

CHAPTER 24

General Patton hadn't done well during peacetime, and neither did Dilan. Outside the OR, clouds filled his mind like Portland's fog. Sure, the adrenaline rush of a good operation was rewarding. And now, finally, he was earning money—good money, enough to start paying off some of his student debts, and with more money on the horizon. Average pay for an American neurosurgeon was upward of $600,000 a year. But he was lonely and depressed. The adrenaline rush of a successful surgery always wore off. Then you were back in that murky place.

Now that he was an attending physician, he was responsible for his patients' trajectories, including any work that he directed residents to do. As an attending, he spent more time with patients and their families, which created more challenges. You wanted to teach your patients about the procedure and their chances—lay out all the options and decide together what to do. But you had to do that without freaking them out. That was no small job, considering that you might have to remove half of a patient's skull and dig through his or her lobes. Before complex surgeries, he spent days thinking about what might go wrong. If he lost a patient, he spent weeks imagining whether he could have done something differently.

The fog lifted when he was in the OR. The operating light cranked out more than eighty thousand lumens, similar to the mid-afternoon sun. This bright light turned the brain's veins and tissues into a Grand Canyon of reds, whites, and pinks. A needle-thin artery might rupture and shoot a jet of crimson until you brought the suckers to bear. But at least it had clarity, like the air and red earth around Haydom in the dry season.

He found his mind trying to conjure the colors of Haydom: the piles of pale-green scrubs he and Mayegga dug through before operations; the yellows and whites of the eggs and potatoes in *chips mayai*; the browns of the acacias that floated like smoke in the valley below the hospital. When memories weren't enough, he put on his brown Keen shoes, still stained red. To preserve the dust, he didn't wear them in the rain. When he put them on, he instantly felt more grounded.

Memories of Tanzania spilled out during breaks. "I was so unplugged there. No cell phone, no Internet. All I had was my *Lonely Planet* and what I could fit in my backpack," he told an assistant one day at lunch. "I was happier in those six months than I'd been in the rest of my life."

At night he paced. His house had a wraparound porch. Head down, eyes seeing but not seeing, he walked from one end to the other for hours. Haydom wasn't in his life anymore, gone like his relationship with Jenny, and it all felt like death and its stages: shock, then bargaining. *Maybe I can find some way to get back to Haydom.*

Then anger.

He remembered how the Tanzanians stood in the rear of the radiology room, how he asked the medical students to move to the back but how some sat in the front the next day. And then new medical students arrived, and he played musical chairs again, saying, "We're just visitors; they will be the ones who take care of patients long after we're gone. They're the most important people in the room."

The porch's old wood sagged in spots. Pacing over these dips, he remembered the derogatory way foreign doctors talked about the Tanzanians.

"They just don't care," one had said.

"They're useless," another told him.

The human brain craves patterns. *Who was useless?* Foreign doctors had poured into Haydom for decades, but to what end? People were still dying every day because the hospital simply didn't have enough trained doctors, midwives, and nurses.

He stopped now and then to lean against one of the wooden columns. *Look at the whole picture. Abnormal or normal?*

Abnormal.

You would never have enough visiting doctors to fill the demand. People would always be dying because of this failure. And failure meant you had to learn from your mistakes.

This is bigger than Haydom. How big? He had no idea.

Few of the big players in global health were talking seriously about the shortage of doctors, much less the dearth of surgeons. None of the United Nations Millennium Development Goals mentioned the shortage of surgeons and other skilled health-care workers. The United Nations' 356-page update in 2005 didn't use the words *surgery* or *surgeon* once. When the Bill & Melinda Gates Foundation unveiled grants in 2005 for the "grand challenges in global health," none went toward increasing the ranks of surgeons. Dilan wouldn't know until later, but another surgeon was about to make a critical discovery that would clarify the seriousness of this shortage.

His name was Haile Debas, the avuncular director of the University of California Global Health Institute. Like Dilan, Haile Debas was an immigrant, in his case from an area in Ethiopia that eventually became Eritrea. "I'm living proof of the brain drain from Africa," he once said.

Debas moved to Canada as a young man to earn his MD at McGill University, then eventually to San Francisco. In time he became the university's chancellor. Throughout his remarkable career as an academic surgeon, he found his mind drifting back to the country of his birth and how he might help his people.

He had a chance in 1991 when Eritrea won its independence. He crafted a plan to build a medical school but then set it aside when Eritrea's new president decided to postpone elections for "three or four decades." When the World Bank asked him to do a report about global surgical issues, he wondered, *Exactly how bad is the shortage on a global scale?*

He knew anecdotally that it was a huge problem. All you had to do was count the number of surgeons in low-income countries. In the mid-2000s, Malawi had only fifteen surgeons to treat its twelve million people; Sierra Leone had fewer than ten, and only one was under fifty years old; Tanzania had about seventy surgeons for its forty million people.

But what was the true impact of this shortage? Did more people die and live with disabilities because of this gap? If so, how many? When Debas searched for hard data to answer these questions, he found almost nothing. He would have to come up with his own numbers.

He and several colleagues collected information about the world's health problems, from traffic injuries to tuberculosis. Then they examined whether surgical intervention could have healed these injuries and diseases. In 2006, they published their discovery: Eleven percent of the world's "global burden of diseases"—deaths, injuries, diseases, and disabilities—could be averted or treated with surgery.

Eleven percent was a stunning number when spread across a growing population of 6.5 billion people. It showed that if the world had more surgeons, millions of lives would be saved. Traumatic injuries alone killed five million people a year, more than malaria, tuberculosis, and HIV/AIDS combined. Half a million women a year died in childbirth, often because no skilled doctors were available to stop hemorrhages and other complications. Countless others died of burst appendixes, infected gallbladders, and hernias; cancer patients died sooner because simple tumors weren't removed; people with cataracts went blind.

Debas knew the 11 percent figure told only part of the story. The number didn't take into account affordability, transportation to and from health centers, and many other factors. But it was a starting point, something that exposed the seriousness of a problem that had been hidden in plain view.

Dramatic as it was, Haile Debas's finding generated little interest outside a small group of health leaders and researchers. Brian Mullaney, cofounder of Smile Train, would say later that the shortage of surgeons was "the biggest global health problem no one's heard of."

During breaks between cases, Dilan took the aerial tram to his office in the skyscraper below the hospital. There, he sat in his chair and paced in his mind.

The global health picture?
Abnormal.

Life expectancies in the poorest countries were still half the level of the richest. Thousands of doctors flew to poor countries to do short-term missions, but instead of helping countries become more independent, the opposite had happened. Haydom Lutheran Hospital wasn't an aberration; it was the norm. Forty percent of all the health-care providers in sub-Saharan Africa were faith-based organizations. Parts of South America and Asia were just as dependent on outside groups. And Haiti—it was the poster child for the missionary industrial complex. As many as ten thousand NGOs were on the island. People called it the Republic of NGOs. The United States pumped $300 million a year into Haiti, all through NGOs.

Sure, it was important to spend billions of dollars on AIDS, tuberculosis, and malaria. But he remembered his conversations with Oystein Olsen in Haydom—hospitals shouldn't just focus on specific diseases; they should strive to be competent in all areas, including surgery. Dilan looked at the walls. No family photos. No pictures. It looked as if he hadn't moved in. He had lots of ideas floating about in his mind. But what could he do about them? He had a floor-to-ceiling window. Outside, the sky was bright white, like the frosted pane on his office door, no definition at all.

During one of these midmorning breaks, he met with a researcher who did work in South America. Naturally, he told her about Tanzania, and how he taught Mayegga brain surgery. Mayegga was saving lives now, he said. But Mayegga was just one person. For Tanzania to truly move forward, it needed hundreds of Mayeggas. And, man, he told her, he really wanted to go back.

"I'm so homesick," he said.

Dilan had left the frosted door to his office open. Kim Burchiel, chairman of the neurosurgery department, walked in.

"Dilan, you need to find some structure to what you're doing," he said in a terse voice.

"What do you mean?"

Burchiel was a lean man, athletic, with a thick head of gray hair and a gray goatee. He was among the world's most respected experts in the surgical treatment of neurological pain.

"You've got to be more organized. If you want to make a difference in Tanzania, get some people to help you. You can't do it just by yourself. Otherwise, it will distract you from your job in Portland."

By that, Dilan knew he meant "your real job."

CHAPTER 25

The brain has more neurons than the Milky Way has stars, and in the course of your life, these neurons form millions and millions of circuits. Each circuit performs a task. The neuroscientist David Eagleman calls these subroutines "zombie systems," because most operate as if on autopilot. These zillions of subroutines help us do everything from form words to pick up a spoon, or after years of sleepless nights in the operating room, peel apart a patient's temporal lobes. The subroutines work with great efficiency, which allows the brain to save energy for more complex tasks, such as asking directions in a language you don't know, or thinking about the criticism you just got from the department chairman. The subroutines make up a massive chorus, nearly all of which plays behind the curtain of consciousness.

And like any large choral group, some subroutines work well with each other, some sing off-key, and some compete for the lead. With so many subroutines, the brain is as messy as a democracy, what David Eagleman calls a multitudinous "team of rivals." But intelligence and wisdom are rooted in this raucous network of competing and congruent circuits. This conflict is our strength. Our inner wiring, vibrating with rivalry, allows us to weigh complex ideas, choose right from wrong. It is the electrochemical architecture of our conscience.

Like the brain, human society has its own multitude of subroutines. When it comes to helping the poor, the missionary model held sway for centuries, itself a mix of yearnings to conquer new land, convert others to different beliefs, help those in need, and live lives of adventure and meaning. The missionary model has modern variants: the Marshall Plan after World War II; John F. Kennedy's Peace Corps; and more recently, the emergence of short-term missions. Like the brain's subroutines, these paradigms compete for hegemony, creating a chorus in the world's conscience. The noise grows especially loud when the subject of foreign aid comes up.

On one side are people like Jeffrey Sachs, the economist from Columbia University and author of the best seller *The End of Poverty.* Sachs believes that poverty is rooted in geographic isolation, epidemic diseases, poor governance, and unfavorable climates for agriculture. These factors prevent poor countries from reaching even the bottom rung of the global economic ladder. Until they have a firm grasp of that first rung, they will be stuck in "a poverty trap." His prescription is a "big push" in the form of foreign aid.

Sachs and others have plenty of examples of how foreign aid has lifted millions out of poverty. On a global level, vaccination campaigns have all but wiped out smallpox. In Tanzania's case, the government in 2001 used aid to help double its education budget, and enrollment in primary schools went from 60 percent to 90 percent in five years. With the right kind of aid, Sachs and his supporters say, ridding the world of extreme poverty is possible only when wealthy countries make the effort. In *The End of Poverty*, Sachs concludes, "Let the future say of our generation that we sent forth mighty currents of hope, and that we worked together to heal the world."

Others argue that foreign aid is a trap of its own, that life expectancies in many poor countries have barely gone up despite push after push. Dambisa Moyo, a young Oxford-trained economist from Zambia, argues that average per capita incomes have stagnated or gone down in Africa since the 1970s. "Has more than $1 trillion in development assistance over the last several decades made African people better off? No," she writes in her book *Dead Aid.* She has particular contempt for "glamour aid." She told *Newsweek,* "If there is a criticism I would level against celebrities—they have tended to perpetuate negative stereotypes. They always tend to portray Africa as a horrendous basket case. They want to portray the war, the poverty, the disease, the corruption. As an African, I'm tired of it . . . Taking a picture with a starving African child—that doesn't help me raise an African child to believe she can be an engineer or a doctor."

She and others argue that aid crowds out local investment and encourages corruption and conflict as political and military elites try to protect their aid sources. Aid brings humiliation instead of dignity; it perpetuates dependency. Foreign aid, Moyo writes, "has been, and continues to be, an unmitigated political, economic, and humanitarian disaster for most parts of the developing world."

A few months after Burchiel's lecture, Dilan had stopped pacing. Now when he went onto the porch, his mind was filled with ideas. Burchiel was right. He was disorganized. His thoughts about Tanzania were like those nurses and residents in the OR during his first operations, fluttering about instead of flying in formation. Now his thoughts were lining up.

When it came to foreign aid, the question shouldn't be whether to help. The desire to help others was a noble goal. Rather, it should be, what is the *best* way to help?

Transferring skills had to be part of the answer. Improving human capacity. Humanitarian efforts too often focus on *stuff*. Sure, many low-income countries desperately need more equipment and medicines. Tanzania had just three CT machines. But isn't it a bigger injustice to have three brain surgeons for an entire country? Yes, teaching has the power to change people's internal wiring, help them do things they never thought possible. And teaching is a universal value, as basic as a father teaching a son to tie his shoes. Which means it can be a unifying force.

In the brain, an idea forms when a signal shoots through a neuron at two hundred miles per hour toward a sac of molecules. When the signal hits that sac, it pushes the molecules out of the neuron, like a gust pushing through an unlatched door. This happens over and over, lighting up different parts of the brain until you think of a good place to get pizza or decide to create an international health program.

That's what Dilan would do—set up a program to help doctors teach in East Africa. "Teach first" would be its guiding philosophy. *Teaching has to be the overriding priority*, he thought, *or the paradigm isn't going to change*. Some of these "teach first" trips would be short, but it was just the beginning. They would focus on neurosurgery but expand to other specialties. The idea was simple: If you could teach brain surgery in the African bush, you could teach pediatrics, internal medicine, obstetrics, and anesthesiology. In the end, those specialists would save more lives than brain surgeons. But brain surgery would be the vehicle to expand people's perceptions about what was possible.

He called the program Physician Training Partnership. *Partnership* was an overused word in medicine and business, but forging real bonds with institutions and people in low-income countries had to be more than a euphemism. The old colonial paradigm had to go. His missions would be about teaching, first and foremost, with the goal of creating medical peers—partners.

Now that he had a vehicle, he could invite others to climb aboard. He brainstormed with assistants, neurologists, medical students, anyone who showed a spark of interest. His enthusiasm was contagious; word spread through OHSU about his program, then to neurosurgery departments in Colorado, North Carolina, Massachusetts, and then to Europe. Colleagues and friends began making plans to travel to Tanzania to teach instead of treat.

Through a friend, he met Robert Hamilton, a former Peace Corps volunteer in Ethiopia in the late 1960s who had a PhD in anthropology. He'd worked in marketing, in sales, and as a stockbroker. Now in his sixties, Hamilton had his own NGO called Progressive Health Worldwide that distributed medicine in India. "You know, in the end it's all about investing in people—in the Tanzanians," Dilan said. "And the investment would pay off when those Tanzanians teach other Tanzanians." Hamilton found himself taken by Dilan's charisma and message. He agreed to be the director of Dilan's new group. And to reduce the red tape, they put Physician Training Partnership under the umbrella of Hamilton's existing NGO.

Dilan found volunteers in Colorado and Portland to work on logistics. Dilan's mother helped out with bookkeeping and organized the first fund-raiser. During a conversation between surgery cases, a colleague suggested he find a grant to study Mayegga's surgical performance.

Of course!

If he wanted to show that it's possible to teach brain surgery in low-income countries, he needed real data on mortality and complications. He assumed that Mayegga's brain surgery patients had fared well. But he didn't know for sure. And a grant would come with another benefit: his contract in Oregon allowed only two weeks of vacation. A grant might be a ticket to a longer stay in Haydom.

With a few phone calls and e-mails, he convinced a medical equipment company to contribute $10,000 annually for a neurosurgery resident's monthlong stay in Haydom and the costs of renting a vehicle to find Mayegga's patients. It didn't take long to find volunteers for the study.

"Yes, you're coming to Tanzania," Dilan told one of them, Rachel Chard, a first-year medical student. He looked her in the eye, and she felt instantly connected to what he was doing.

"Dude," Dilan told Jonah Attebery, another OHSU medical student. "Haydom is awesome. You'll love it." Attebery made plans to go.

Dilan would join them later that summer as they wrapped up their hunt for Mayegga's patients.

He kept telling himself, *This is huge. Here's a problem that's killing people, and almost no one is paying attention to it.* The shortage of doctors was like a big subdural hematoma. If you ignore it, the patient dies. How can you stand there and do nothing?

He discovered something about himself as he worked on his program: unlike the adrenaline high after a challenging surgery, this feeling lasted. In fact, working on an important global health problem was the perfect counterweight to the pressures of neurosurgery. Doom and danger stalked him inside the hospital, but when he thought about Tanzania, he felt a sense of possibility, not despair.

Solutions—that's where the energy was. Get cancer, and you'll find little hope by concentrating on the disease. But think about treatments and, boom, your mind moves toward what could be; you'll talk about options, you'll talk with others about what to do, which could trigger more ideas, move more neurons. Then you can take action, move forward. Ideas and action were hope's sparks and tinder. *A chance to cut is a chance to cure.*

Dilan's forte was his ability to bring people together and brainstorm. But he was a reluctant leader. He believed that if an idea has merit, then people should naturally rally around it. They should bring their own talents and ideas to bear. During Physician Training Partnership meetings, Dilan talked about how he wanted people in his group to collaborate like researchers—as a group of equals.

But that didn't fly with some senior doctors. A neurologist named Mary said, "We're not completely equals. You and I are faculty members, supervisors. We should take care of our students, and the students should be accountable to us."

"That's your opinion," Dilan said and moved on to another subject.

When people asked him about logistics of getting to and from Haydom, he gave vague answers tempered with encouragement. "You'll figure it out. You'll love it."

Part of him wanted volunteers to experience the awakening that came with discovering something on their own. If he played tour guide, he would cheat them of that joy. Another part of him didn't like lazy thinking, an echo from residency. Despite growing tensions in his young group, more people made plans to join him in Haydom that summer in 2007: Elisa, a chief resident from the Barrow Neurological Institute in Arizona; Mary, the neurologist; Amy, an office assistant in Portland; Lori, a photographer and filmmaker; and Robert Hamilton, the new NGO director. Yes, his life was moving forward again. Kim Burchiel had been so very right, which stung. He hated to admit that Burchiel was right about anything.

They'd gotten off to a bad start when he surprised Burchiel about his plan to take six months off and go to Africa. Dilan heard from other colleagues that Burchiel was fed up with his global health work. Well, he was fed up with Burchiel's desire to control his life.

Burchiel was correct that his work in East Africa was time con-suming. When he wasn't in the OR, he was on the phone with doctors and residents, saying, "You should go, but only if you want to teach. If you teach, your impact will be huge."

But he pulled his weight in the operating rooms. And his global health work only enhanced the university's reputation. Colleges and teaching hospitals across the world were scrambling to establish beachheads in distant lands. Students expected to have overseas ex-periences during medical school. Oregon Health and Science Uni-versity had only just begun to create a comprehensive global health center. Physician Training Partnership could help put Burchiel's department and the university on the cutting edge of an important international health issue—the shortage of surgeons.

Then again, his criticism of traditional short-term missions could create some headaches for his boss. One of the most prominent neurosurgery NGOs was a group called FIENS, short for Founda-tion for International Education in Neurological Surgery. FIENS had organized surgical missions to low-income countries since 1969, and a few members had done impressive and lasting work. Merwyn Bagan, a New England neurosurgeon, had spent years in the 1990s teaching in Nepal, which had just one local neurosurgeon at the time. David Fairholm, a surgeon from British Columbia, moved to Taiwan in the late 1970s to train local doctors. Before he arrived, the hospital did about 140 neurosurgeries in a year. When he left in the early 1980s, its local doctors were doing more than two thou-sand a year.

Fairholm and Bagan had gotten it right; they made long-term commitments to teaching. But they were ahead of their time and their success stories had been overwhelmed by the growth of short-term medical missions. Dilan had learned that most FIENS members now did brief trips and then went on safaris or moun-tain hikes. These doctors had good intentions, but as far as Dilan was concerned, they perpetuated a broken model. Now, here he was in Oregon, fresh out of residency, talking about how more experienced neurosurgeons were doing harm. Burchiel couldn't be pleased about that.

And Burchiel had already lectured him about how budding neurosurgeons were supposed build their practices, invent new surgical techniques, write grant proposals and research papers, work just as hard as they had in residency.

Dilan was trying to do all these things. He had long considered himself a researcher as much as a surgeon. Before his arrival in Oregon, he had written or cowritten more than thirty academic papers. His work at the University of Virginia on microbubbles had been on the cover of the *Journal of Neurosurgery*; if he and other scientists were right, someday you might attach tumor-destroying medicines on the surfaces of tiny bubbles, shoot them into the bloodstream, and then pop them with ultrasound blasts when they reached their targets—surgery without a blade. He'd turned in a National Institutes for Health grant proposal, but Burchiel sat on it for weeks.

He sent Burchiel an e-mail about his $10,000 grant from the medical equipment company. He expected a congratulatory reply but got a terse note instead: You didn't ask for my approval. We need to talk.

And Dilan had thought, *Yes, we do.*

CHAPTER 26

One of Burchiel's assistants held up a box of tissues when Dilan walked into the office suite. "You might need this," he said with a smug look on his face.

Dilan ignored him and took a seat at a round table in Burchiel's office. His left hand rested against the side of his face, index finger pointing up toward his temple, his thinking pose.

Burchiel sat on the opposite side and began with a list of complaints: Dilan was disorganized in his work at the hospital, just as he was disorganized with his work in Tanzania. The microbubble grant application? It wasn't ready, and he wouldn't sign off until it was in better shape. And that grant to look at Mayegga's work? Bad move. In the future, he wouldn't be allowed to talk to representatives of medical equipment companies. From now on, everything would go through him.

"And forget about your work in Tanzania. You can't go."

"On my vacation?"

"Dilan, I can't let you go. That's not why I hired you."

Dilan took his hand off his face.

I can't go to Tanzania?

Burchiel sat back in his chair, waiting for Dilan's response. Seconds passed, then a minute, one of his long silences. Jaw clenched, he began:

"You know this is my first job, and I honestly didn't know what to expect as an academic neurosurgeon, but here's my conclusion: I think it's like dating. And just like dating, sometimes it takes three dates to know whether you're compatible or not. This is our third date. And, no, we're not compatible. I think it's time for me to resign."

Burchiel furrowed his brow.

Dilan added, "I'd like to have twenty-four hours to think about it before letting you know for sure, but I think it's time for me to find a place where I fit better."

Dilan stood up. Neither made a move to shake each other's hand.

His eyes narrowed into gun slits as he walked out the door. He turned toward the assistant but decided not to say what was going through his mind: *Fuck off, I just fired the boss.*

Nearly all his mentors called that night.

From Harvard, Arthur Day said with a chuckle, "Dilan, what the fuck? You asshole. What are you doing?" He said he'd gotten a call from Burchiel. "He really wants you to stay."

From Virginia, John Jane also suggested that he reconsider, but added, "Yeah, that's the problem. I didn't train you to work for a chairman. I trained you to be the chairman."

Others left messages. He dodged their calls. He had made his decision.

No one was going to tell him to set aside his work in Africa. It was too important to shut down. And no one was going to tell him how to run his life.

He would take a financial hit, for sure. He still had more than $160,000 in student debts and another $14,000 of debts on his credit cards. He had no job, no relationship. But he felt a sense of relief bordering on happiness, as if he'd been released after being locked in a dark room.

He put what few belongings he had in storage. Maybe this was what he'd been looking for all along: no ties, no responsibilities, a backpack full of clothes, and a plane ticket to Tanzania.

Then just before he left, Jonah and Rachel sent him an e-mail from Haydom. They were done with their research. He printed out the attachments and glanced at the numbers.

"Ooof."

He stuffed the pages in his backpack as if he'd opened a door, seen something horrible, and slammed it shut: a peek and shriek.

But he'd seen enough to get an overall picture. And it wasn't good. No, it was a disaster.

CHAPTER 27

Dilan had made it seem so simple: just go to Haydom, find the records of Mayegga's patients, and see how they were doing. No sweat. It'll be awesome.

But when Jonah Attebery and Rachel Chard finally made it to Haydom, they discovered that the operating theater's records were missing. No one had an explanation. "It sometimes happens," clinicians said. They would have to find the patients' names some other way.

They found a few in a green hardbound ledger in the hallway and more in the radiology, anesthesiology, and billing departments. They eventually compiled a list of more than fifty names.

Except they had no addresses, just their names, their villages, and in a few cases, the names of elders. They sat with Emmanuel Mayegga in the dining hall and spread out a map. Fortunately, Mayegga had a sharp memory and remembered many cases, including details about where the patients lived. Only one patient was from Haydom proper; the rest were spread across the plateau. At least three were nomadic Maasai, who could be almost anywhere. Their plan ended up as simple as Dilan made it out to be: just go to the villages, ask people if they knew where so-and-so lived, and go from there. As Jonah looked at the list, he saw needles and haystacks.

Jonah, a tall man with a thin, dark beard and glasses, had gone on overseas church missions in high school. Even then, he felt a little unsettled about their usefulness. Later, in medical school, he read *Mountains Beyond Mountains*, Tracy Kidder's book about Paul Farmer, a medical anthropologist and epidemiologist who co-founded Partners in Health.

In Farmer's mind, those with means had a moral duty to liberate the poor from their suffering. Farmer spoke of "stupid deaths"— deaths from diseases that could be easily prevented with safe and affordable medicines. He used the term "structural violence" to describe how poverty and injustice fostered diseases that killed people just as horribly as bullets and grenades.

Inspired by Farmer's quest for medical justice, Jonah had spent the previous summer in Uganda at a small clinic. To his surprise, he found that local medical officers expected expats to bring donated medical supplies and do most of the work. Two weeks into his visit, someone asked for his shoes. It was as if they had been taught to be helpless. Jonah left Uganda feeling that the dependency on foreign doctors was destructive to the Ugandans, and that he was a coconspirator in this cycle. But Dilan's enthusiasm could be irresistible, so now here was, in Haydom, which was as awesome as Dilan had said.

Mornings typically began in the dining hall for breakfast with the Norwegians. Then, with Phillip, their Tanzanian translator, they piled into a gray Toyota truck. Since Tanzania was a British colony, people drove on the left, which meant Jonah had to learn how to shift with his left hand. Phillip sat in the middle, and Rachel squeezed into the passenger seat. They stowed a couple of extra gasoline cans in the back and were on their way.

When they reached a particular village, they stopped and asked bystanders if a certain patient lived nearby, often giving rides in exchange for directions. Sometimes, four or five men climbed into the back.

With Jonah and Rachel asking questions in English, Phillip searched for expressions in Iraqw, Swahili, and a few other local languages to convey the meanings of *unconscious* and *muscle twitches*. They gave basic exams, which triggered laughs when they asked patients to say, "Ahhh," and even more laughs when Phillip relayed questions about incontinence. A large group often gathered during these examinations, and Jonah wondered what would happen in an

American town if two strangers showed up and asked random questions about a person's urination patterns.

On one search they found a man whose wife had died at the hospital and who seemed to have something on his mind. He invited them into his hut, and they all sat on the dirt floor. With Phillip translating, they learned that his wife had been to the hospital for a biopsy and died a short time later. No one at the hospital had told them what was wrong with her brain or why they did the biopsy. He believed she had died from the biopsy, and that this is just what happened in a poor country.

Rachel told him his wife hadn't died from the biopsy, that she'd developed glioblastoma, the most common and invasive form of brain cancer. Even with surgery, it's impossible to remove every star-shaped cell of these tumors. She said that people in the United States also contracted this cancer and died. He seemed surprised by this, and she saw his facial muscles relax. Cancer had taken his wife's life, not some unqualified clinician. For Rachel, this was a lesson she vowed to remember for the rest of her medical career: education could heal.

Some days they struck gold and found three or four patients. Other days, they struck out. It didn't help that some of their targets thought they were bill collectors. A few protective neighbors gave them wrong directions to steer them off course.

On a trip to the eighteenth and final village, they found a *mama* and her infant. The baby had one of the makeshift IV-tube shunts. The hut was made of mud and sticks and was about four feet high inside. Goats were in the next room. The child was swaddled in rags. The mother handed the baby to Jonah, who suddenly found himself overwhelmed by emotion. *What a gift it was to hold such a fragile life.* This was why he went into medicine.

Jonah asked the mother if she had any questions.

With Phillip translating, she asked, "What's in my child's head? And can we take it out now? Can I do it myself?"

Jonah shuddered. He imagined the woman taking a knife and cutting out the shunt. Shunts were permanent. Pull one out, and the baby he was holding would die from an infection or bleeding. He and Rachel tried to explain the purpose of the shunt. Later, his uneasiness turned into anger. The mother clearly had no idea what had happened to her child. Why was she allowed to leave the hospital without knowing more about the shunt procedure?

Done with their visits, they tallied and indexed the results. They calculated complication and mortality rates and compared them with rates in the United States and other areas of the world.

When they finished they thought, *This is bad news.*

CHAPTER 28

Dilan squeezed into the cramped airplane seat, right side, by the window and near the back. Portland to Minneapolis to Amsterdam to Arusha—twenty-eight hours sandwiched into the cheapest seat he could buy. He wore the same cotton khaki pants he had during his first trip. He wore the same brown Keens. He stuffed his backpack into the overhead compartment. The results of the study were in an outside pocket.

The jet climbed, and the pilot turned off the seat-belt sign. The flight attendant passed with drinks. No thanks. He wanted some uninterrupted time to dig into the data. He looked out the window.

The hills below were shaped like the brain's sulci and gyri, the wrinkled folds that made up the frontal and temporal lobes. The lobes were really sheets of cortical neurons. The wrinkles were the secret to our intelligence. You could pack more of these sheets into the skull if you crumpled them like a newspaper wad. Dilan wasn't feeling so smart as he thought about those papers stuffed in his backpack.

As the jet flew east, the green folds around Portland gave way to harder slopes: the Sawtooths, the Bitterroots, their peaks as sharp as molars. He stood up when he noticed the flight attendant had finished drink service. He opened the overhead compartment and removed a sheaf of papers. He avoided eye contact with the passengers next to him. He sat down and hunched over the data, left elbow on the edge of the table, left hand rubbing his forehead.

He read Jonah's and Rachel's e-mail again, then moved to the attachments. A table showed the mortality rates of Mayegga's operations.

Shit, Dilan told himself. *This is bad.*

He turned to the complication rates. *Shit.*

He leaned back in his seat, looked out the window. It was getting dark, but he could still see jagged rows of mountains below.

Scrap the program. Now.

Admit your failure. Figure out why it went wrong. Learn from your mistakes. It's the only way you move forward. Forgive and remember.

How had Mayegga failed? How did I fail Mayegga?

He dug into the data again. Of the fifty-one neurosurgery patients Jonah and Rachel had identified, fourteen had died. Terrible.

And it didn't make sense.

He'd been there with Mayegga for many of these procedures. Mayegga's work was excellent. And he had seen some of these patients post-op. Most seemed to do well afterward.

His eyes settled on the dates of the procedures and the dates when patients died.

Interesting. Some patients died weeks after the operations.

He looked at the causes of death. Of the fourteen who died, six succumbed to malaria, pneumonia, and other causes unrelated to the surgeries.

Malaria? You didn't contract malaria from an operation. Those deaths weren't related to Mayegga's work. The pneumonia cases were less clear. Patients who stay longer in a hospital tend to pick up pneumonia and other diseases. Poor follow-up care and infection-control practices could have caused some of those deaths, but not Mayegga's hands.

He looked out the window again. The plane had cleared the Rockies. They were over flatlands now, probably Montana, heading toward the Dakotas.

What about the high number of infection-related deaths? Poor surgical techniques could increase the odds of infections. Of the eight remaining deaths, five were caused by infections. He studied another table: many of the infection-related deaths and complications involved hydrocephalus cases.

Then it hit him.

It's the shunts.

Or rather the IV tubes—they used IV tubes instead of normal VP shunts, his idea. Some patients had returned because the shunts developed blockages. Blockages often lead to infections. In several cases, Mayegga had to replace these shunts, another opportunity for infections and complications. Clearly, the IV tubes hadn't worked as well as he'd hoped.

That stung. Yes, those patients would have died anyway without surgery, but the makeshift tubes had just prolonged their pain. They had done harm.

At least the data showed that Mayegga's surgical performance was solid. *OK, maybe this isn't so bad after all.*

In fact, if you factored out the IV-tube and malaria cases, Mayegga's numbers were comparable to or better than hospitals in East Africa with experienced surgeons. He sat back in his seat.

Actually, this is pretty good news.

He put up the tray table and locked it in place. He placed the papers in his lap. He stretched his legs under the seat in front of him.

Am I manipulating my interpretation of the data to make myself feel better? Am I trying to make Mayegga look better?

He went through the data again, then put the papers back in a folder and stuffed it all in the seat pocket. As the flight attendant passed by, he asked for a soda. He put down the tray table; he felt the forward momentum of the jet.

No, factor out the shunts and nonsurgery-related deaths, and Mayegga's performance was solid. He had learned how to do brain surgery.

This is real.

In Haydom they spotted each other on the dirt path between Radiology and the dining hall. Mayegga beamed and gave him a hug. Mayegga wore a white doctor's coat over a blue plaid shirt. A small spiral notebook and pens were stuffed in his lower left pocket.

"Come, come. I want to show you." He took Dilan's hand. "I've been doing things."

In the radiology office, Mayegga sat at a computer and called up a CT scan. Dilan grimaced: the skull was shattered on the right side, and the pressure had moved the patient's entire brain to the left. The evidence was in the bent midline and the shadows of the ventricles. It was a huge subdural hematoma.

The patient's name was Petro. He'd been drinking with some friends near the village of Bashay when someone smashed his head with a stick. He arrived at the hospital barely conscious and paralyzed.

Mayegga clicked his mouse and another CT appeared—Petro's brain a day after Mayegga operated on him.

The skull's shape was virtually normal. The fluid was gone; the brain had sprung back to where it was supposed to be.

"Incredible," Dilan said. "You did that?"

Mayegga nodded. "Yes, of course."

Dilan leaned forward toward the computer.

"Man, you can't get any better than this. It's a perfect result. I can tell you this: you wouldn't see such a good result in a North American hospital."

Mayegga grinned again and said something in English that Dilan couldn't quite make out. Something about a patient. Dilan guessed, *Maybe he wants some advice about another patient?* Mayegga seemed unusually excited as he took Dilan's hand again.

He led him out of Radiology to the operating theaters. Clinical officers had small offices in an alcove near the entrance. Mayegga motioned for Dilan to take a seat in his office. Dilan sat next to an exam bed with a wrinkled green sheet. The office's white walls were bare except for a folding calendar turned to the month of July. A wooden desk was in the corner with an old Dell computer and a few papers scattered next to it.

"Wait, let me show you this man."

A few moments later, Mayegga reappeared with a man who looked to be in his early thirties. He was dressed nicely in dark green pants, black loafers, a green V-neck sweater, and over the sweater, a banana yellow jacket.

"Dr. Dilan, this is Petro."

"Wait, is this your patient? The one with the big subdural?"

"Yes, it is him!"

Mayegga asked Petro to turn his head. Petro's hair was cut short, but Dilan could barely make out a semicircular incision.

Mayegga took his seat at his desk with a look of utter satisfaction.

To Dilan's eyes, Petro looked stone-cold normal. After such a devastating injury? Unbelievable.

Neurosurgeons have a simple test to detect lingering brain damage: Ask patients to extend their arms with the palms up, as if catching raindrops. Then tell them to close their eyes. If the patient's brain is damaged, one arm will drop.

Dilan asked Petro to hold out his arms and close his eyes. He looked at Petro's hands.

Steady as oak.

"I can't believe it," Dilan said. "This is the same one we saw in Radiology?"

"Yes, yes. I'm telling you. He's the one."

"This is beautiful. When did you do this?"

"Two months ago."

"Wow, this is huge." He slapped Petro on the shoulder and slapped his hand into Mayegga's. "You saved his life."

Then Petro turned toward Mayegga. He said no words, but his eyes held Mayegga's for a long, grateful moment.

Dilan thought, *Now we have proof—on paper and in the healed brains of people like Petro—that Mayegga learned brain surgery.* What a wonderful way to begin his visit. And now he would be here for a full six weeks—plenty of time to teach Mayegga to teach others, his next goal, and plenty of time to reconnect with those he met during his first trip. He was back home.

Other thunderclouds were on the horizon, though. Shortly before he left Portland he had gotten a call from Edward Laws, one of his instructors at the University of Virginia and a member of FIENS, the group that sent neurosurgeons across the world on medical missions.

Laws told him that several important African doctors had learned about his work with Mayegga, and they were furious.

"You need to smooth things over," Laws had said, and then suggested he talk with Paul Young, a neurosurgeon from St. Louis.

. . .

Paul Young had done his first medical mission in 1998, arriving in Nairobi, Kenya, with an old operating microscope and seven boxes of surgical equipment. Young had time to do about thirty procedures, but the hospital was filled with brain-injured patients. This meant he had to choose which patients to save and, by default, which ones would die. On his last day, a line of families waited in the hall, pleading, "Please save my son" and "Please save my daughter." Stunned by the need, he returned to Kenya over and over, growing more convinced with each visit that medical missions would never fill the demand.

Young also was a member of FIENS, and in 2005 he began working with Moody Qureshi, a Kenyan neurosurgeon, on a curriculum to teach neurosurgery. They would instruct only qualified East African MDs—not clinicians.

So, when he reached Young, Dilan half expected to be chewed out. He described his work with Mayegga, and soon they were finishing each other's sentences.

"Don't worry. Just keep doing what you're doing, and tell them your story," Young said, giving him the names of Qureshi and Abedi Kinasha, one of Tanzania's three brain surgeons.

Now that Dilan was back in Tanzania, he was determined to tell his story to these two men. But how?

He set aside the question as he waited by the library steps before morning report. He stood on the red dirt, still feeling joyful about Mayegga's success with Petro. Surgery could be miraculous. And now Mayegga, not some *mzungu*, was the miracle worker. He looked east toward the cottages.

The canopies of the jacaranda trees were speckled with light. He could see the foreign doctors following the red paths toward him. Out of the corner of his eye, he spotted Oystein Olsen, the medical director, who was staring toward the cottages. Someone was coming up the hill: a tall woman in white.

   Then Dilan's eyes focused on the woman. She took long strides. She wore a white coat and white pants; she held her head high. After she passed under the jacaranda trees, the rising sun struck her blonde hair, lighting her in a silhouette. Then he saw her face, her smile. Suddenly he felt a stillness inside, and in this space nothing but light.

CHAPTER 29

That morning Carin opened her eyes as the sunlight struck up the chorus of birdsongs. Yes, she was in Tanzania, not the Netherlands, or still dreaming. At this hour, the sun was the color of untarnished copper. She listened to the birds as she gathered her clothes and stethoscope. Tasks left undone in the Lena Ward flooded her mind, and she flew out the door, stuffing her stethoscope in her lower left pocket. She strode up the hill toward the library, head held high, back straight, arms swinging, steps so forceful that she could easily walk out of her clogs.

In morning meeting she saw the new group of Americans. They wore long white coats with their names embroidered in fancy blue script. They had a confidence about them, an intensity she'd seen in other surgeons, which could be a problem here . . . well, anywhere. In the Netherlands, she had found many neurosurgeons to be arrogant and aloof. Would they boss the Tanzanians around?

Later, in the radiology meeting, she studied them more closely. The Americans stood in the rear of the room, and they talked easily with the Tanzanians, though the tall one with the shaved head seemed more serious, as if lost in thought. He held his chin high, which accentuated his height. His arms were crossed.

In the front, Dr. Naman sat at a desk and prepared the X-rays and CT scans. As he was about to begin, the tall American raised his voice.

"So, I think it would be good if the foreign medical students in the front rows gave their seats to the Tanzanians. These are the people who will be here after we leave."

Carin held her breath. She studied his body language. He was still; his legs were set wide. He didn't look angry, but he wasn't happy either. She was glad he spoke up. She also hadn't liked how the medical students took those front seats.

The silence held for a moment, but then the students stood and offered their chairs.

Dr. Naman pulled up a CT scan of a patient's skull.

"Patient is thirty-four years old from Singida," Naman said.

The American spoke again, "Yes! A beautiful scan!"

"Dr. Dilan!" Naman said, turning and nodding toward the American. Heads turned again.

"So, this patient," Dilan said, "who wants to give it a try?"

Silence.

"Normal or abnormal? You have a fifty percent chance of being right."

"Abnormal!" a clinical officer replied.

"Excellent, doctor!" Dilan pointed his finger to a young clinical officer. The clinician had high, raised eyebrows that gave his face a look of permanent surprise.

"Now, can you point out what's abnormal?"

Dilan handed a long wooden stick to the clinical officer, who drew a big circle around the entire brain and then threw a furtive glance at Dilan, who nodded slightly. The clinical officer turned back and made a smaller circle, then looked at Dilan again to see if he was getting warmer.

"There you go. There's the tumor. See, you don't need me at all!"

Dilan explained what the tumor was and how it affected the brain's anatomy.

"So, Dr. Mayegga, you and I are going to remove this tumor. What do you think?"

Mayegga stared at the scan for a few moments with a serious look, deep in thought, then said in English, "Sure, it is not a problem."

The meeting broke, and the clinicians and doctors fanned out. Carin headed toward the Lena Ward, thinking for a moment about the American. He seemed different from the surgeons she knew in Holland. He led from the back of the room, shifting attention away from him and toward the clinician and Mayegga. More like a coach than a player. And he had called the clinical officer doctor, just as she did.

These thoughts burned brightly for a moment, then like embers, drifted away amid brighter flames: the children in the Lena Ward. So much to do. She told herself to just think one thought.

OK, go to Angela.

"Daktari Carin! Come back! Pili just stopped breathing!"

She spotted Nurse Angela's urgent wave. Carin rushed into the ICU, third door on the right.

Pili was two years old and had pneumonia and meningitis. A nursing student hovered over mother and child, holding an oxygen bag about ten centimeters away from Pili's pale face, which did the child no good whatsoever. Carin realized the nursing student had no idea how to give oxygen. *But look how she's trying. She just hasn't been properly taught.*

"You did good work starting the resuscitation. Let's put her on the table."

The color in Pili's face grew grayish blue.

"Here's how you place the mask. You press it firmly to the child's face." Carin moved her other hand to the bag and gave it a gentle squeeze. "See how the chest rises. You can really see the lungs filling with air. And you can hear it, too. Now, you try it."

Carin moved quickly to intubate the child as the student took over. Together, they watched the color return.

"You just saved her life, well done!"

"*Asante,*" the student replied—thank you—her face full of pride.

Angela, however, looked grim. Only three nurses were on duty that night, not nearly enough to take care of 150 children, much less one struggling for every breath.

"What will we do?"

Carin was struck again by the sadness in Angela's eyes. The day before, Angela had said, "No matter how hard we work. They die anyway." Would Pili be next?

"Who do you have in the evening shift?"

"Malia and Restituta."

"Restituta!" Carin said. "Is she the one who wants to specialize in pediatric nursing?"

"That's her," Angela said.

"Good, let's teach Restituta."

Restituta had a short but muscular frame, high cheekbones, and eyebrows shaped like the wings of a diving hawk. She spoke quickly and clearly and in a formal way that Carin loved. When Carin took her to see Pili, she said, "Well, Daktari Carin, this is a very seriously ill patient! She is deeply unconscious to major touch and loud speech and not making any breathing efforts herself."

"You're absolutely right, Restituta! I can't tell you how happy I am that you're on call."

"Why, Daktari?"

"Because I think with you, Pili has a chance to survive."

Restituta looked straight at the child, frowned a bit, as if calculating Pili's odds.

"I think so too, Daktari! She has a strong body, and she did not come in too late. We just need to help her breathe until the antibiotics work optimally. That will be . . ."—she counted the hours in her head—"at three o'clock tonight."

"Well, there you go!" Carin wanted to hug her.

For an hour, they went over proper ventilation techniques. Before she left for the night, Carin wanted to leave Restituta with one more lesson.

"We should try our very best tonight, but if we do that and Pili still dies, then we can say we did all we could do. Sometimes, even when we try our best, we fail."

On her way back to her cottage, Carin passed a mortuary and said a silent prayer for Pili and Restituta; the sun was low, and the air had cooled. She thought about the Americans, and she felt a sudden urge to ask the tall one with the shaved head about what happened that morning. She turned toward their guest cottage.

Mary, the neurologist from Oregon, met her at the door. She was in running shorts and a T-shirt. Elisa, the chief resident from

Barrow Neurological Institute, sat on a chair in a living area. And Amy, Dilan's former assistant in Portland, stood by holding a camera with an enormous lens. Carin heard the sound of someone taking a shower, then a call from behind the door: "Sorry, bad hair day!"

Mary rolled her eyes. "He's such a goofball."

"An unemployed goofball!" Amy added, without explaining.

Now dressed, Dilan walked out and flopped onto the couch, legs spread wide, arms behind his head. After a bit of small talk, Carin turned to Dilan.

"You have a different approach toward the Tanzanians than other people here."

He smiled and grabbed a beer. "You know, it's something that I had to learn. In America and Europe, we're taught that the patient deserves the best treatment possible. We've trained to become the best. And then when we come here, we jump in like superheroes. You can see it all around, how the visiting doctors just take over."

Carin nodded. "Yes, that bothered me as well. But it's hard to not do things yourself."

"Yes, but in the long run, it's better to teach," Dilan said, gulping the last of his beer. "You'll help more people that way. It works in neurosurgery. Emmanuel Mayegga is living proof of that. And if it works in neurosurgery, it will work in pediatrics and family medicine."

Carin slept lightly that night, worrying in her half-sleep about Pili. The next morning she filed into the library. *Someone would have called if Restituta had run into trouble. Or maybe not, if Pili had died.*

A clinical officer recited a roster of new admissions and then a list of those who had died, name, age, cause. Pili wasn't mentioned. When he finished, Carin blurted out, "Pili survived?"

"No news."

"That's good news then?"

"No news," he repeated.

She rushed to Lena Ward. Restituta was gone; her shift had ended. But there was Pili's mother, caressing her child's cheek. Pili's eyes were half open, and she was breathing on her own.

CHAPTER 30

Dilan had never seen anyone quite like Carin. Her hair glowed in the sunlight; her skin had the silver shine of Haydom's dry-season moon; she walked lightly, as if about to bound. He thought to himself, *She just exudes energy.* She seemed to care about everyone, from the children in Lena Ward to the older man hanging X-rays before radiology meetings. No other foreign doctor helped that guy, him included. Neurosurgeons often managed feelings like strict parents, given all the death and risks of their field. In Carin, he saw someone who allowed compassion to flow through her without inner calculations. One day he watched her try to revive a dying baby. She pumped on that baby's chest for an hour, long after most doctors would have given up. She gave every ounce of herself. He saw the shadows in her face after she turned away from the child's limp body. He thought, *She's a better doctor than I am.*

Because she was there, he loved Haydom even more than before. He told himself, *I've got to find a way to get back after this trip.* As he walked across the hospital compound, he felt as if he were floating in a swift current, something larger than himself.

But now and then another subject disrupted this flow: What about the East African neurosurgeons, the ones who were pissed off about his instruction of a clinician?

He needed their blessing to continue. He'd made his mind up about that. His work was about creating medical peers, not forcing his will. If they told him to stop teaching, he would do that. If they thought he was doing something wrong in Haydom, he'd let it all go.

Paul Young had said, "Just tell them your story," and he took Young's advice. He invited Moody Qureshi, the Kenyan surgeon, and Abedi Kinasha, the Tanzanian, to visit Haydom. He half expected them to decline, given that traveling to Haydom from Nairobi and Dar es Salaam took at least a day or two each way. But to his surprise, they accepted.

Now they were somewhere between Arusha and Haydom in a Land Rover with Robert Hamilton at the wheel.

On his way back to Haydom, Robert Hamilton pressed the brake pedal. Nothing. He pressed harder. It went to the floor. Hmm. Hamilton found he could slow the Land Cruiser by pumping the brakes, shifting into low gear, and applying the hand brake. So he didn't mention anything to Moody Qureshi and Abedi Kinasha, who chatted in English and Swahili in the seat behind him. But then the brakes went out completely.

There was no place to stop for repairs. So he broke the news.

"My goodness, did I hear this man correctly?" said Moody Qureshi, the Kenyan, glancing at Abedi Kinasha, the Tanzanian.

They continued through the Mbulu Highlands, with its switchbacks and forests of eucalyptus, and then onto the plateau. Hamilton knew that just before Haydom, the road curved steeply down a hill to a single-lane bridge over a deep ravine. If another car or person or goat was on the bridge, then something or someone wouldn't make it across.

Seven hours passed. As they neared that bridge, Hamilton asked whether they should stop. After a brief discussion, the neurosurgeons agreed: keep moving forward.

A group waited at Mama Naman's restaurant in the space normally reserved for the pool table. Mama Naman had cleared the room and placed a row of small tables end to end. She draped the walls with white sheets and blue *kangas*. The smell of roasting goat meat blended with wood smoke.

Carin joined the group. She had no idea the two African surgeons were upset with Dilan. As far as she could tell, everyone was simply looking forward to dinner and beers. In the distance, she heard the Land Cruiser and its shifting gears. And then it appeared, moving slowly on the rutted road.

The truck stopped with a final lurch of the hand brake. Everyone cheered. Moody Qureshi and Abedi Kinasha climbed out and stretched their legs. Moments before, they had plunged toward the narrow bridge with nothing but a hand brake. Fortunately, no one was on the bridge, and they rumbled across without incident. Qureshi began describing Hamilton as "the man who saved our lives."

Soon they were at the table drinking bottles of Sprite and Kilimanjaro beer. Moody Qureshi wore a dark sports coat and slouched a bit in his chair as he told the story of their journey. Abedi Kinasha sat next to Qureshi and encouraged everyone to hoist a few more beers. Mayegga quietly sat across from them in a gray cardigan sweater. Carin's flip phone pinged with a text: a diabetes coma emergency in Lena Ward. Her face grew serious. Dilan noticed.

"Are you on call?"

She chuckled. "Yes." She was the ward's only doctor; she was always on call.

Dilan's eyes followed her as she stood and walked toward the gate. Then he turned his attention to Qureshi.

"I'm really glad you made it here in one piece," Dilan said. "And you got to see how far away we are from everything." He lifted his beer. "Here's to surviving your trip." He wasn't entirely sure his teaching program would survive the next day.

The next morning before the presentation Kinasha and Mayegga did a VP shunt procedure—Haydom had proper shunts now—and Kinasha showed Mayegga a new way to manipulate the catheter. Mayegga took over at one point, and afterward Kinasha had said, "Well done." Then it was time for the meeting.

In the chapel, chairs were rearranged to face a white wall, which would be used as a screen. A projector sat on a table. Light streamed through tall, narrow windows, making the first slide a bit dim. Mayegga and Rachel began with the vitals: the hospital was very difficult to reach, as the doctors themselves had experienced the day before, but it was the primary hospital for a growing population of 1.7 million people in the region.

They clicked on other slides that showed the results of Jonah and Rachel's quest a few weeks before—Mayegga's record as a brain surgeon.

Dilan glanced at Qureshi and Kinasha. These were the damning numbers he'd seen on the plane. No signs of emotion on their faces.

The final slide showed Mayegga teaching Jonah a VP shunt procedure, a Tanzanian teaching a *mzungu* medical student. Above the photo was a question: "The Future of Neurosurgical Care in Rural Tanzania: Training of non-MDs as an intermediate step?"

Qureshi stood first. He wore a gray sweater over a white T-shirt and held a piece of paper in his right hand.

"Mayegga's work is impressive," he said, shooting his left hand out to punctuate his points. "An assistant medical officer doing brain surgery! Quite an accomplishment!"

And yes, the shortage of neurosurgeons was a severe problem throughout East Africa. The status quo wasn't acceptable. And for this very reason, he and several other East African neurosurgeons had begun work on a training program with Paul Young of St. Louis. They were drawing up a two-hundred-page curriculum that could be used at universities in Tanzania, Kenya, Uganda, Rwanda, and other parts of East Africa. He liked Dilan's "teach first" approach; transferring skills and knowledge was the only way to bridge the surgical gap between the First and Third Worlds.

"But," he concluded, "we can't do this by training AMOs to do neurosurgery. They're not doctors."

Qureshi returned to his seat, and Kinasha took the floor. He was a thin man with glasses. He wore the same tan coat he'd had on the night before. He kept his hands in his pockets. He spoke so quietly at times that Dilan had trouble hearing him.

He agreed with Qureshi; Mayegga's work was indeed impressive. He had seen him operate with his own eyes. Mayegga was saving lives. The shortage was severe in rural areas, and it also was a serious problem in Tanzania's large cities. Patients who survive a subarachnoid hemorrhage sometimes were flown to India for cerebral angiography or even surgery. His voice rose.

"In Dar es Salaam, there are just three of us!" Yes, Mayegga did not have a medical degree, "but if we don't train AMOs, people will die."

Qureshi dug in: "I can tell you that we cannot train non-MDs to do neurosurgery in Kenya."

"We're not Kenya," Kinasha said again, flashing a wry smile at Dilan, then raising his voice again: "This is Tanzania!"

Dilan sat back for a moment and thought, *Here are two African neurosurgeons debating how to solve a serious health problem. That's success in itself.* And also, *What an interesting display of how Kenyan culture differed from Tanzania's.* Kenyans were often said to be louder and more aggressive than their neighbors. Even some Kenyans described themselves as East Africa's New Yorkers. Among Africans, Tanzanians were often thought to be more reserved and more likely to work by consensus instead of competition. The contrast reminded him of Canada's complex relationship with the United States.

But he knew they had all arrived at a pivot point.

He interrupted, "That's the beauty of this. We don't have to train non-MDs in Kenya. We can do as Moody says—advanced training with physicians in Kenya. And in Tanzania, we can train AMOs. Our main goal is to transfer knowledge and help East Africa become independent of foreign doctors. But we want to do it as partners. We want to work with you. And we absolutely don't want to do it if we're not wanted." He smiled at Qureshi to let him know that he had heard him. "And we definitely don't want to train AMOs in Kenya."

When the meeting broke, Qureshi took Dilan aside. "This has been a paradigm shift for us." He confessed that most of his training and clinical work had been done in Nairobi and other urbanized areas. He hadn't fully realized the impact of the surgical shortage in the bush until he took that long trip to Haydom. He invited Dilan to visit him in Nairobi and learn more about the work they were doing with Paul Young.

Later, during dinner, he pulled Dilan aside. "And by the way, you do realize that we were going to sue you."

. . .

Dilan took stock: A few weeks before, he was on a plane to Africa, thinking about scrapping his NGO. Now he was laying the groundwork with other African neurosurgeons for a region-wide push to train more neurosurgeons. He felt like doing a double fist pump.

But something else had become clear after the two neurosurgeons left Haydom: he had put his friend Emmanuel Mayegga in a difficult spot.

Moody Qureshi's concerns about teaching AMOs were valid. Mayegga might know how to do brain surgery, but the government could easily ban AMOs from doing it in the future. He had promised Mayegga that he wouldn't get into trouble.

Now he wasn't so sure he could keep that promise.

CHAPTER 31

Emmanuel Mayegga passed under the pale orange glow of the lamp by the hospital gate. A few steps away from the light, and darkness wrapped around you like a *shuka*. Steep gullies lined both sides of the road toward Haydom town, and you had to pay attention so as not to fall into one. But away from the light, you could hear your footsteps more clearly. It was as if the darkness and dirt soaked up the background noise of the day. It allowed the voices in Mayegga's mind to grow louder. *Should I go to medical school?*

He followed the road to town and Mama Naman's. These days he usually arrived before Dilan, which gave him time to drink a Kilimanjaro and watch the news on the TV over the bar.

Sure, he'd shown everyone that he could do brain surgery. He was saving lives. But he had heard what Moody Qureshi said—how they would *never* train AMOs in Kenya to do that. If that was the case, wasn't it just a matter of time before Tanzania did the same?

He went over it in his mind. Without a medical degree, people outside Haydom could question his qualifications to do neurosurgery, maybe even other kinds of surgeries. Maybe, in the future, doctors in Haydom would say, "You're not a doctor. You can't do surgery at all."

And there were new doctors on the way to Haydom. Tanzanian doctors. Fresh out of medical school, thanks to the second Dr. Olsen and his wife, Mama Kari. In the early 2000s, the Olsens had begun to identify promising secondary school students. And instead of sending these students to clinical officer school, as they had done with him, they sent them directly to medical school. Over time, a few had chosen to stay in the cities. It was wrong of them, Mayegga thought. They were thunder without rain. But he also understood. Everyone knew you could make more money working in Dar es Salaam or Mwanza. If given a choice between money for his family or a promise to the hospital, he might choose the city.

Some of these sponsored students kept their promises, though. In fact, the first of these young MDs, Emanuel Nuwas, had just returned to Haydom.

He knew Nuwas. He was a sharp and confident young guy. He'd grown up in Getanyamba, a village on the plateau about eight kilometers from Haydom.

And just a year behind Nuwas in medical school was Hayte Samo. Hayte came from the area near Mount Hanang and was about to become a doctor against particularly long odds.

Nuwas and Hayte wouldn't have his years of clinical experience. And they wouldn't know how to do the surgical procedures he'd learned over the years. But they would have something he didn't: a medical degree. And that would trump his clinical training every time.

He was sitting on one of the bar's couches when Dilan walked in wearing an easy grin. To Mayegga, Dilan seemed unusually happy. Without saying anything, they automatically moved to the back patio. Baba Naman joined them and took his usual seat at the end of the table. Mayegga sat facing the horizon, now black. Naman took scotch; Dilan and Mayegga had Kilimanjaros. Light came from bare bulbs behind them in the bar.

"What to do, Dilan?" Mayegga said. "What to do?"

Dilan sat for a long moment. Over the years, when he'd come to a crossroads, he'd found it helpful to ask himself what regrets he might have if he didn't take a certain path.

"So, what would it be like if you didn't go to medical school?" Dilan said.

"Well, then there would be doctors coming in, and I would still be an AMO. So I might not be able to do as much as I can do now."

Mayegga's face looked as if he were in physical pain. Younger doctors would be his bosses. His mind moved to other thoughts.

It often took two days to travel between Dar es Salaam and Haydom, which would make it difficult to return during short breaks. What about Samwayma? She was pregnant with their second child now. And his son, Godwin, and his father?

"Do I leave my family? It is five years. Five years in Dar es Salaam!"

And he would be twenty years older than some of the other students. He hadn't done any serious book learning for years.

"I'm already old!"

"You're doing neurosurgery in this hospital," Dilan said. "If you can do that, medical school is going to be a piece of cake. But, yeah, five years is a long time to be away from your family. That's a lot to give up. I'm not sure you should go."

They sat quietly for a while.

"So, if you do go to medical school, what would that be like?" Dilan asked. They'd gone through the regrets. Now the possibilities.

Mayegga took a swig.

"With a medical degree, I could do surgery in Haydom." He could save lives in the future, as he had done in the past. And, he would likely get a small salary increase, which would help his family. He would move forward in his career, be a doctor, not just in the eyes of those in Haydom but far beyond its horizon. He could teach what he had learned from Dilan.

Dilan said, "I'll tell you this: you have the talent to be a world-class surgeon. With a medical degree, you could be the chief of surgery here at Haydom someday."

Dilan turned to Baba Naman and asked what he thought.

"I think you should go. You're still young. What's a few years?"

Mayegga drained another bottle.

And then he had another thought: What about all the patients who needed him? Once he left, who would care for those babies with hydrocephalus?

Nuwas had shown some interest in neurosurgery; perhaps he could teach him.

"What to do, Dilan? What to do?"

.   .   .

Emanuel Nuwas had always wondered how those hydrocephalus shunts worked. How did you move the fluid from the brain all the way into the abdomen? No one had taught him the answer in medical school.

But then Mayegga had shown him: Just drill a burr hole in the skull, slip the tube in above the ear, and work it down the neck just under the skin. Then shimmy it down the chest until it reached the abdomen. The body absorbed the fluid nicely there. He'd thought, *So simple!*

Nuwas had puffy cheeks and eyes that sometimes narrowed into a mix of concentration and mirth. While Mayegga's fingers were long and thin, his were short and bulbous, like sausages. His voice was softer than Mayegga's, except when he preached during *Sala*. He raised his voice just a few decibels, but something about that amplification and his confidence lifted his words to the rafters.

Soon after his return to Haydom from medical school, he'd asked Mayegga to teach him various surgeries. Mayegga was grateful to have a little backup. Then Mayegga had taught him to do shunts in the brain. And now the American neurosurgeon named Dilan was showing him other procedures. And they were excellent teachers. First they put him on the "doing" side of the operating table, even though he was just observing. The next time they did the procedure, he did most of the work. Mayegga and Dilan scrubbed in but sometimes even stepped into the hallway. And the third time? Dr. Dilan might say, "Hey, I'm in the cottage, call me if you have a problem." He'd felt something inside surge. A neurosurgeon trusted him, a young doctor just out of medical school!

Emanuel Nuwas had always been a confident person, someone who ran toward action instead of away from it. Like those twisters on the plateau. When he was young, the dry-season winds lifted the red earth around his family's *boma* and sent it spinning. He ran straight into them, and it was such a wonderful feeling because they pushed you around, lifted you up. Sometimes you felt as if you could fly.

His parents scolded him for doing that, of course. It was dangerous and bad for your lungs. And he was supposed to be the responsible one, the oldest of nine children, the one to carry the family's weight.

His mother, an Iraqw woman, taught him that when you said bad things, you should spit. This was a reminder to think before you said something negative. And she told him to taste the words as well. If they tasted bad, you knew that you had said something wrong. She encouraged him to go to school, once saying, "If I had gone to school, I think I might have done something great." And she taught him to greet the morning sun. Traditional Iraqw culture held that the sun was both man and God. Praising the sun was a sign of thanksgiving and respect, a time to think of what the day's possibilities might bring.

His father was Datoga, a good-natured man who drank too much. Sometimes he drank so much *piwa* that he had to sell the family's cows to pay debts. He returned to the *boma* late at night, yelling in a happy way most of the time but of little use when the sun rose. And so it was up to his *mama* to plow the small *shamba* field. And because she was in the field, Nuwas cooked for his younger brothers and sisters and cleaned the wet cattle manure from the room next to where they slept.

As with Mayegga, he'd lived in a chest-high hut surrounded by a circular fence of thornbushes and brush. He trapped dik-dik with sisal ropes and chased monkeys away from the maize. As he grew older, he woke up at five in the morning, collected firewood, and set off for Haydom, the earlier the better. You got the best prices for firewood then. When he wasn't selling firewood, he fetched pails of water for *mamas* in Haydom, trotting down a hill to the river below the bridge. A twenty-liter bucket might get you enough for a pencil or small piece of soap.

He was an excellent student, and when he graduated from primary school, he gave a presentation on gastrointestinal issues. At the end he asked, "Any questions?" Among those in the audience were the second Dr. Olsen, his wife, Mama Kari, and Baba Naman. "Such a smart and confident boy," they all said to each other.

They would sponsor his secondary schooling and then his training in medical school. And now, with his MD, he was back in Haydom, learning from Emmanuel Mayegga and the American neurosurgeon, plunging into people's brains as he had into those red and brown twisters.

CHAPTER 32

After six weeks Dilan was on his way back to the States, but he wouldn't be gone for long. He would make sure of that. His global health work was gaining momentum: He'd built friendships with East Africa's most influential neurosurgeons. And Mayegga was teaching Nuwas brain surgery.

Nuwas was the real test of his program's true potential. You could teach someone brain surgery, but if the teaching stopped there, then the impact was minimal.

Still, he wasn't so sure about Nuwas. Dilan could see that Nuwas was smart, and that he had a bit of the swagger he saw in surgeons. But he might be a bit too confident. A chance to cut was a chance to cure—and also a chance to do more harm.

Most of all, he felt the clock ticking because of Carin.

She had no idea that he wanted to be with her, but he told himself, *If I'm gone for six months, she'll be with someone else. Three months away, and I'll still have a chance.*

On his last day, he mixed good-byes with promises. "I'll be back in three months," he told the Namans, Mayegga, and then Carin. And by the way, he added, he was thinking about buying some land in Haydom. Would she care to join him for a look?

Late that afternoon they piled into the gray Toyota pickup that Jonah and Rachel had used in their hunt for Mayegga's patients. Dilan drove off the road by the hospital's gates onto a thorny area just below the hospital's fence. The land fell steeply to a riverbed. The wind blew hard as they jumped out of the truck. Carin walked to the edge of the hill and crouched on her knees. He joined her.

"Do you really think you will live here?" she asked, staring at the horizon.

"I'm not sure," he replied. "I'm different here. I love the dirt, the essence of things. But I don't want to be just another *mzungu* who comes and goes. Hey, so I'll be back in November."

"Good," she said, and took one last look at the horizon before she stood up.

Back at the hospital, Dilan parked near the dining hall and loaded his bags. Carin lingered as he took his time saying his good-byes. He turned to Carin. "I'll be back in November," he said again. And then they shook hands.

CHAPTER 33

Skilled surgeons don't stay unemployed for long. Not in Africa. Or in North America and Europe. Although the surgical shortage is at crisis levels in Africa, wealthy countries have their own doctor deficits, though in the United States, the wounds were self-inflicted.

In the 1980s trade groups and researchers incorrectly forecast a doctor surplus. Fearing a glut, Congress, in 1997, all but capped the number of residency slots. The predictions turned out to be wrong.

Forecasters failed to take into account that doctors were retiring sooner than expected, many because they were fed up with long hours, lawsuits, and insurance hassles.

Further, demographic shifts toward families with two working parents made the old workaholic Harvey Cushing model increasingly less tenable for those who wanted to see their children grow up.

Then, in 2003, new work rules limited residents' workweeks to eighty hours—the same work rules that Dilan and his colleagues ignored at Virginia. Most residents didn't share this defiance, which meant teaching hospitals suddenly lost an enormous amount of relatively cheap staffing. Meanwhile, North America's population had grown larger and older, creating more demand.

By the mid-2000s, researchers believed the United States was facing a deficit of ninety thousand doctors by 2020, including a gap of forty-six thousand surgeons and medical specialists. Similar demographic forces were affecting doctor-patient ratios in Canada and the United Kingdom. Throughout North America surgeons were in particularly short supply in rural areas. Nine hundred of America's three thousand rural counties lacked a single surgeon. Critics called these rural areas surgical deserts.

To keep their health care systems afloat, the United States and other Western countries had long drained doctors from poor countries. Some had criticized the practice. As far back as 1967, Walter Mondale, then an American senator from Minnesota, said it was "inexcusable" that the United States should "need doctors from countries where thousands die daily of disease to relieve our shortage of medical manpower." A 1974 congressional report noted that the current US policy was widening the gap between rich and poor nations and warned of the "great potential for mischief in the Nation's future relations with the LDC [less developed countries]."

But the brain drain continued. International recruiting companies sprang up across the world, luring health care workers from India, Nigeria, Haiti, Pakistan, and other countries with critical shortages. An Indian physician called it "the great brain robbery." More than 260 American companies specialized in recruiting foreign nurses. Recruiters advertised salaries that might seem extraordinary in poor countries and offered to pay legal and immigration costs to move them. These recruiters took in as much as $55,000 in profits per placement. Forty recruiting companies admitted they were helping doctors and nurses leave disadvantaged regions.

It was a silent aid program from the poor to the rich. Many governments in Africa subsidized the educations of their doctors. So when their newly trained doctors left, their investments exited with them. The United States saved $846 million in training costs by luring doctors from nine African countries, one study found. The United Kingdom was an even bigger beneficiary, saving $2.7 billion. In 2001 British health policymakers issued a code of conduct to discourage recruiting in low-income countries. But more than a decade later, hospitals were still hiring three thousand doctors from abroad every year, including physicians from Syria and the Sudan. The United States had more than 5,300 doctors from sub-Saharan countries, such as Liberia, Sierra Leone, Tanzania, and Kenya. All told, one out of every four doctors in the United States had been trained outside the country.

Dilan's skills in cerebrovascular surgery were in particularly high demand. Of 3,700 neurosurgeons in North America, only 25 percent specialized in cerebrovascular work. And fewer still did aneurysm microsurgery. Worldwide, strokes are the second leading cause of death after heart disease; half a million people die from ruptured aneurysms every year. If you survived the rigors of a neurosurgical residency, you had job security for as long as you could competently hold a scalpel. For Dilan, the question wasn't whether he would find a new job, it was where.

Within weeks he had two offers: one from the University of Colorado Health Sciences Center in Denver and another from the Medical University of South Carolina in Charleston. Both were solid institutions in beautiful cities. He decided to bring Carin into the decision-making process. He shot her an e-mail about the offers. She answered:

> Your job . . . hmmmm lucky bastard! What about the people? Any
> particularly nice ones? You are perhaps a blunt surgeon but also a bit of
> a social animal in the end. Good luck, Ca.

Go where you like the people best—good advice. But he liked people at both places. In Colorado, they had already put his name on an office door. They were thrilled about his work in Tanzania. Same thing in Charleston, minus the plaque on the door. But in Charleston the department's cochairman, Sunil Patel, had been born in Tanzania of all places. From Tanzania, Patel's family had moved to Zambia, and then eventually South Carolina, an immigration story not so different from his own. And the clincher: Charleston was much warmer than Colorado, more like Sri Lanka and Africa.

Before he started, though, he would spend another six months in Haydom. Six months for sparks to hit tinder. It was a gamble. Carin might not be interested in him, of course. And he knew he was hurting his career no matter what happened between them. He'd just learned that MUSC was creating a new cerebrovascular program. If he started work in Charleston immediately, he would probably run it. But six months away? Another ambitious neurosurgeon would likely step in. A Harvey Cushing type wouldn't let such an opportunity go.

He composed another e-mail.

Dear Carin,

I can barely sit still in my seat! Exactly one more week to go and then I am on a plane coming back to Tanzania. Feels like I FINALLY get to go home again and for a nice long uninterrupted time. Everything here is tidied up—got my contract signed and squared away, all the loose ends tucked in.

He ended by mentioning that before arriving in Haydom he was going to Arusha first to buy a truck. Mayegga and some other friends would meet him there. They would be at a hotel called Dragon Pearl.

Would she come to Arusha and help him choose a truck?

He pressed send.

CHAPTER 34

Yes, Carin had said, she would meet him in Arusha. She wasn't sure why he needed her help to buy a truck. It didn't make sense, and maybe that's what clinched it. But instead of riding with Mayegga and his friends, George and Samweli, she would fly there a day early with Tor, a handsome Norwegian missionary pilot who was clearly interested in her.

Tor picked her up on the airstrip in Haydom, and soon they were high above the plateau's *shambas*. Near Mount Meru, Tor detoured through Arusha National Park and flew just above the treetops.

In the air, Tor was an artist. He used the plane's wings to draw circles in the updrafts and downdrafts. He was sensitive, cutting the engine so they wouldn't scare the animals. But on the ground, Tor was different, or perhaps who he truly was. Driving through Arusha, he growled and cursed at pedestrians, forcing them out of his way, a pushy *mzungu*.

Carin breathed a sigh of relief when he dropped her off at the Flying Medical Service compound. It was part farm, part dormitory, and for Carin, a sanctuary because of its director, Pat Patten. Pat was a Catholic priest with a gray beard, glasses, and more knowledge about the Maasai than a PhD. Pat sat back like a father listening to a daughter's travails, then asked with a friendly grin, "And you're going to Arusha tomorrow to pick up another guy?"

Dilan, Mayegga, George, and Samweli spent the night at the Dragon Pearl, a hotel with white columns, a red tile roof, red Chinese

lanterns, and a friendly manager named Louie. The next morning
Dilan sat on the porch with a plate of bread and jars of peanut butter
and jelly. He wore the khaki pants he'd worn on his previous trips,
a blue-and-white shirt, and a green corduroy sports jacket. He'd
shaved his head. He looked down the driveway, which was lined
with orange birds of paradise.

A small Japanese SUV appeared. Pat Patten was at the wheel.
Carin was next to him.

He stood up and trotted down the porch steps. He watched
Carin give Pat a hug inside the car. She climbed out and turned
toward him . . . and burst into a grin.

Eight years before, Carin had waited for a train in Amsterdam's
Central Station with a crumpled piece of orange paper in one hand
and a pen in the other. Images of men she knew floated through
her mind like confetti in the wind, and she'd had a sudden urge to
gather these bits in one place.

Men will fall in love with me, but why don't I fall in love with them?
OK, let's get away from specific men, look at the overall picture. What
are the qualities I most like in a man? What would the perfect husband be
like? She picked up her pen and used her knee as a desk: He would
be religious, but in a genuine way, spiritual. He would be friendly
and wise. She scribbled as the train came and went. He would be a
man who believes he's part of something bigger, someone solid and
peaceful, and strong in a protective but gentle way. She'd kept that
orange sheet of paper for years, thinking that if she met a person like
that, she would know in a flash.

After saying good-bye to Pat Patten, she saw Dilan walk down
the porch with his open, childlike face, his big wide eyes. She saw
him stop at the base of the stairs and wait, still smiling.

She knew. He was the man she'd written about so long ago.

CHAPTER 35

Medical school?

Emmanuel Mayegga wondered at the thought. *How can I leave now?* Word had gotten out that Haydom Lutheran Hospital could do brain surgery. Patients were coming from as far away as Moshi, the city by Kilimanjaro, and Mwanza, the city by Lake Victoria. Depending on the mode of transportation—ambulance, bus, bicycle, or foot—it could take eight hours to several days to get to Haydom from these places. One time a patient named Patrice Bura arrived from Tumatti, a village about two hours away. He'd been drinking homemade brew with a group of men when someone accused him of sleeping with his woman, then whacked him on the head with a stick. He walked around in a daze, blood streaming down his face. He had said good-bye to his wife and friends before he lost consciousness.

When Mayegga saw Patrice Bura in the ICU, he knew exactly what was happening inside Bura's head—a classic subdural hematoma. And he knew what to do: first, a craniotomy with the Gigli saw, then cauterize the broken arteries, suck up the excess blood, and close. He operated on Patrice Bura, and within a week, Bura was ready to return to his *shamba* in Tumatti. Mayegga had done fifteen subdural hematomas like this over the past few months, all on his own. *If I leave, what will happen to people like him?*

Then another thought: *Daktari.*

It sounded impressive, but what did he need a medical degree for? He'd removed brain tumors, fixed abscesses. All of these patients would have died without him.

Daktari Mayegga?

As he mulled his future, the baby in Samwayma's belly grew. Then the Short Rains ended, and it was close to the baby's time. Samwayma said she wasn't feeling right, and he rushed her through the hospital gates.

He asked a nurse to do an ultrasound. Check for a fetal heartbeat.

The nurse prepared the machine. Mayegga watched the transducer move across his wife's abdomen. His heart sank.

Samwayma delivered a lifeless body, a baby girl. The umbilical cord had wrapped around her neck.

The days afterward passed in a blur.

Medical school? He told himself, *I don't want to set foot in a hospital ever again.*

Baba Naman sat in his plastic chair on the back patio. Sometimes when Naman had a long day at the hospital like this, Mama Naman put her hand on his shoulder and said, "Husband, I have not seen you for so long," and Naman's cheek pads rose like a young boy's.

Mayegga took a seat next to him. Naman could see the pain in his eyes. Over beers, Mayegga erupted about the hospital, the news of the world, different things; Naman knew what had happened to Mayegga's family, knew that Mayegga's raised voice was just steam; best to let it vent and then steer Mayegga gently toward a decision. They went over it:

What about the patients he would leave behind? Well, now that he'd taught Emanuel Nuwas, that problem had been solved.

The money? Oystein Olsen had said the hospital would sponsor his training.

"Baba Naman, should I really leave my family behind for so long?"

Naman answered, "Life has its ups and downs. Don't worry too much about the lows, and celebrate the highs, because neither will last forever. You should go. Your fingers were born to do surgery."

Mayegga drained another beer and looked at the horizon.

. . .

He decided later that Baba Naman was right. Dry seasons came and went; some were longer than others, but the rain and its blessings eventually returned. Nuwas and Hayte were part of a cycle: new MDs were coming with the credentials he lacked. He knew brain surgery, but his skills were worthless if he couldn't use them—like that old broken Gigli saw Dilan found when he first arrived.

He would keep moving forward, as he had from the *boma* by the rocks so long ago; he would move to Dar es Salaam and try to become a doctor.

CHAPTER 36

On the driveway of the Dragon Pearl, Dilan and Carin felt as if they had formed a single circuit; energy flowed between them in a circle, brightening every thought about the present and what might follow. They didn't know each other that well, or at least the details of their pasts. But they would learn those specifics as they drove back to Haydom and she confessed how she cried often, how she had felt so awkward and lost when she was younger until she had a mission, that she hated the idea of makeup but wore it anyway, and then he had held her and said, "I love all of it, and just so you know, you never have to wear makeup for me." And later on camping trips, when he told her how depressed and lonely he was during residency, how it had nearly broken him until he went to Haydom, where he found a new calling to teach, where he found her. And on sunset walks on the airstrip through the honey light and the first hints of wood smoke, when they reached the spot where he'd spotted the farmer with the wire saw, he turned to her and said, "You know I'm going to marry you, don't you?"

The wedding would be in March, on the airstrip. They left arrangements to Mama and Baba Naman, telling them only, "We want everyone to feel welcome to attend."

"Everyone?" Baba Naman had said. "It's certainly possible."

Within days he formed a committee. The committee sent invitations to surrounding villages. Women sewed dresses and shirts. Naman bought ten huge bags of rice—one metric ton in all. A truck full of potatoes, beans, and cabbage chugged into town. "People love a celebration," he said, "especially when there's food."

As the preparations gained momentum, Carin suddenly had a decision to make. After the wedding and honeymoon, Dilan would head back to the States to start his new job at the Medical University of South Carolina in Charleston.

What would she do?

She had arrived in Haydom with a dream of becoming a missionary doctor like Professor Molyneux in Malawi. But now she had to choose: dreams or love?

She and Dilan talked about options: What if they both stayed in Haydom full time? They quickly ruled that out. Dilan had a new contract and enormous student debts, and come to think of it, so did she—she had spent much of her small stipend in Haydom on patients' bills and powdered milk for the Lena Ward. A financial reckoning wasn't too far off. As for Dilan, she knew he loved Africa but also wanted to make a name for himself in neurosurgery. Ambition was part of his wiring, and he could succeed only in a hospital with advanced equipment and highly skilled nurses. Africa simply didn't have these pieces of the puzzle yet. What if they lived apart and commuted? No, neither wanted to be apart from one another. A more realistic goal, they finally decided, was to someday split their time between Haydom and the United States.

She turned it all over in her mind, usually in the early evenings when they settled on the porch and wrapped themselves in a single blanket. At that hour, the darkening sky had purple hues toward Hanang. The sounds beyond the hospital walls grew louder: barking dogs, children's calls, people talking, a rolling boil of life that felt as warm as their blanket. She would have to leave all this. Just like all the other visitors.

One night in Haydom a few days before the wedding, she found Mama Naman in the restaurant's cook room. Blackened pots and pans were scattered about. Several young employees sat in a corner slicing cabbages. Carin watched Mama Naman sit for a moment as she gave instructions, laughed, and hummed a tune. Flames from the fire cast her face in flashes of orange. Behind her, the room's brown mud walls soaked up the heat.

When Mama Naman saw her standing in the doorway, she stood up, wiped her hands on her apron, and took Carin's head into her hands. She drew her forward for a kiss on the cheek.

"You are too light. The wind will bend you like the grass," she said. "What is bothering you?"

"I'm very happy, Mama. I'm very fortunate to have met Dilan. But life is not all about me. I feel guilty about leaving, about following Dilan."

Mama Naman looked into her eyes.

"Of course you should follow him! My dear, love is the highest value. Everything else comes from love."

CHAPTER 37

The hospital's Norwegian benefactors also faced some difficult decisions, namely, how to keep it afloat.

In early 2008 a Norwegian consultant criticized the hospital for its "high dependency on expats." The consultant noted that the number of paid foreign doctors had risen in recent years, even as the number of local clinical officers and nurses declined. If the hospital wanted to retain Tanzanian nurses and clinical officers, they would have to boost wages. But the consultant dismissed the idea of recruiting Tanzanian MDs, "as these workers are everywhere in scarce supply."

Salary expenses were only part of the problem. The hospital had just begun a bold but costly experiment.

One of the most serious health problems in Haydom and the rest of sub-Saharan Africa was the high number of pregnant women who died in labor or immediately after. Many bled to death because they didn't call for an ambulance, or in some cases, because they were too deep in the bush to get any help at all.

Haydom Lutheran Hospital had an ambulance system, but it charged for this service. As a result, few mothers in labor called for it—just 177 women in 2007. But in 2008 the hospital began offering free ambulance trips for women in labor and no fees for C-sections. It was an instant success.

The number of ambulance calls went from fewer than two hundred a year to more than two thousand. The hospital delivered more than one thousand additional babies. Many of these babies would have been born in huts or small and poorly equipped clinics. In short order, the free trips and C-sections helped reduce the area's maternal mortality rate to among the lowest in sub-Saharan Africa. But each ambulance trip cost about thirty dollars, a bill the hospital simply couldn't afford.

By then its finances were as stretched as an aneurysm sac. The Norwegian government was paying the equivalent of $2 million a year to the hospital, more than half its budget. The Tanzanian government contributed another 10 percent. The rest of the hospital's income came from donations from the Friends of Haydom and patient fees.

To Westerners, the fees seemed unbelievably low. Major operations, such as a subdural hematoma or setting a broken bone, cost seventy thousand Tanzanian shillings, or about thirty American dollars. A CT scan of the brain also cost the equivalent of thirty dollars. An ultrasound cost just six US dollars. But many people in the region made the equivalent of fifteen dollars a week. They simply wouldn't seek treatment if fees were any higher.

This left Oystein Olsen and the hospital's Norwegian supporters with few options. Money from the Norwegian government typically arrived in the form of five-year block grants. As the months passed, the hospital borrowed grant money earmarked for future years, eating its own seeds. And this short-term fix was based on a chancy assumption: Norway would keep sending them money.

CHAPTER 38

On March 22, 2008, Carin opened her eyes as a shaft of sun hit the curtains. On the pillow to her right were scraps of paper. She hadn't slept well. Thoughts about the children's ward had roused her like alarm bells. She'd fumbled for a pen to scribble something down, hoping this would set her mind at rest. But then more thoughts about the children nudged her awake: *Those three newborns were having trouble sucking and swallowing; find out if the new nasogastric tubes are in.* In her half-sleep, she missed the paper a few times and wrote on the sheet. She saw the ink marks and sighed.

She made porridge, filled her pockets with Tanzanian shillings to pay some children's bills, and grabbed her stethoscope and mobile phone. Through an open window she heard the birdsongs, including one that sounded like a pulse oximeter. She looked back at Dilan; his eyelids were motionless, as if he'd sleep another three hours. *Good, I'll have more time.* She might even get back before he woke up. Then it would be off to Mbulu to sign the marriage papers and back to Haydom for the wedding.

In Lena Ward she found Nurse Angela at a desk with her eyes locked on the big black ledger.

Looking up, Angela said, "Oh, you're here! How can you come here on this of all days?"

Carin nodded: I know, I know. Angela pretended to be irritated, but Carin could tell she was relieved. She didn't have enough nurses to do proper rounds.

"Any trouble last night?"

"Oh, yes," Angela sighed. "Elias." The four-month-old boy from Mbulu. A clinical officer had diagnosed pneumonia, and his tiny lungs crackled with every breath.

"Why is he not getting better with the antibiotics?" Angela asked.

Carin put her stethoscope to his lungs. "It's not bacterial."

"Ah, then is it the rainy-season virus?"

"Yes, that one." Technically, it was respiratory syncytial virus, a common bug but one that could be life-threatening for infants. Rainy-season virus was easier to remember.

She went to another room to examine Daniel, an eight-year-old boy with sickle-cell crisis, and then to the ICU for a teen named Christopher. A clinician had wrongly diagnosed him with pneumonia, but Carin had spotted a shadow on the X-ray and determined that it was a bowel perforation, a complication caused by typhoid. Mayegga had operated on him, and now he was doing fine.

"Angela, can we discharge him from the ICU to a room with not so many crying babies?" Christopher looked up with a shy smile and then to the crying baby next to him, a three-month-old with hydrocephalus. A few beds away, Angela nudged a boy with meningitis. He'd been brought in too late. His father was by his bedside.

"*Baba*," Carin said, sitting next to him. "Your boy is still very sick. I'm so very sorry."

She stayed silent, which told the father what would happen.

"But let's not give up on him. Let's do a CT scan now to see if there is anything we can do . . ."

Suddenly a door opened with enough force to sweep sheets of paper from the table across the room.

Dilan walked in, serious, but with a glint in his eye.

Oh, no, Carin thought, *I've lost track of time.* She looked at the children she had yet to examine: premature twins, a boy with a tumor in his throat. She had a stethoscope in one hand and a CT request in the other. She looked at Angela, whose mouth opened wide with shock as Dilan strode over to Carin, hoisted her into the air, and then draped her over his shoulders in a fireman's carry.

"Dr. Hoek will be unavailable for the next month," he said.

Angela clapped and ululated: *Yi! Yi! Yi!* Other nurses joined in. Children popped out of their rooms and cheered. Dilan carried Carin into the hallway and then outside into the sun's embrace.

It was a Datoga custom for men to do this—sweep their wives off their feet and take them to their huts. But she knew the real reason he'd come: A missionary doctor's work never ends. *Thank you for taking on my burden, for carrying me away from my guilt.*

Mbulu was two hours away, although in the rainy season, it might take five or more if a truck got stuck and blocked your way. So they'd decided to sign the papers the day before the wedding, spend the night in Mbulu, and return the next day for the ceremony. Dilan would take their green Land Rover, but she would return by air. She had come to Haydom by air, and she would begin her married life with Dilan the same way.

Leaving Mbulu the next morning, Dilan sped along the muddy and rutted road. Along the way, he passed a bus stuck on a hill, its tires driving deeper into the muck. By the time he made it to the hospital, the Land Rover was covered in brown, and the wedding celebration on the airstrip had begun. Dilan drove the Land Rover to the rear of the hospital. Mechanics raced out like a pit crew and hosed it off. He went with Mayegga and Nuwas to his cottage to change. As he finished dressing, he heard singing in the distance.

He walked out the door and looked up the hill. A group of men and women were heading toward him—the operating theater team. The men wore blue-and-brown shirts, and the women wore similar-colored dresses, all made for this day. They crowded in a circle around him. Cheers went up when Mayegga handed him a long, polished staff:

"Now you have become an *mze*." An older man. "We are your family." He handed Dilan a plaid *shuka*, blue and brown. "And this is the color of our tribe."

"If I'm in your tribe, you'll have to teach me how to wear it."

Mayegga taught him how to drape it over the shoulder and said, "Come, come, it's time."

The Land Rover arrived from the garage, spotless and decorated with garlands of white flowers. Dilan climbed into the driver's seat, and Nuwas and Mayegga slid next to him. The operating theater team broke into song as the truck lurched forward. Men climbed onto the back and stood on the bumper. Its springs sagged from the weight.

Oh, shit, Dilan realized. *I still need to memorize my vows.* He had written them on a scrap of paper ripped from a spiral notebook. He'd thought hard about what he would say. But reading them would be lame. He tried to explain this to Mayegga and Nuwas, who looked confused for a moment and then burst out laughing. Mayegga said, pointing his finger, "You better remember before the wedding!"

The Land Rover cleared the hospital gates. Fifteen people clung to its sides and back. Its engine strained as it climbed the hill. The crowd along the road was five deep. As he neared the airstrip, he heard cheers, then shouts.

"The plane has come! The plane has come!" Dilan pressed the accelerator. Covered in flowers and people, the Land Rover lurched forward.

In Mbulu that morning, Carin tried on her wedding dress for the first time. Her stepsister, Tes, had found the sleeveless cream-colored dress and brought it with her to Tanzania. The skirt had layers at the bottom but was just a simple fabric around the waist. Carin put on earrings with brown glass and draped a sterling silver pendant around her neck.

A Land Cruiser from town arrived. They climbed in for their ride to a nearby airstrip.

The dirt road was slick, and the driver drove quickly.

"Almost there," he said as the Land Cruiser suddenly lost its traction.

"Hold on!" Carin shouted. The car slid into a deep ditch, then tipped over. Its roof dug into the mud.

Carin took stock. She was OK. Tes was OK. The driver was fine but embarrassed.

"*Hamna shida*," Carin said. No problem.

It would take a day or two to get a vehicle free of a mess like this. They would make better time on foot. She climbed out of one of the truck's windows and held her dress up with one hand. She tucked her cell phone between her breasts and bra strap. She took off her wedding shoes and replaced them with walking shoes.

As they trudged through the mud, they heard the sound of the plane. On the side, "Wedding Plane" was painted in bright red. They climbed the hill to the airstrip and waved. "We're here! We're here!"

"The plane has come! The plane has come!"

Dilan heard the chant again as he stopped the Land Rover. The Cessna had landed at the other end of the airstrip.

He climbed out and waded into a sea of color: the green of the grass, fresh and vibrant from the rain; towering white clouds floating in a cobalt sky. Nearby, a large wedding tent made of tree-trunk poles and brown canvas covered a wooden stage. The tent posts were festooned with red, white, and pink balloons. Three cows and at least four goats had been butchered and roasted. Baba Naman had bought enough rice for four thousand people, and all of it had been cooked. Datoga men wore red *shukas* and carried staffs; women held green branches, symbols of peace. Dilan saw members of the area's many ethnic groups: Iraqw, Irambe, Hadza; he spotted his parents, Buddhists from America by way of Sri Lanka, and Carin's tall family from the Netherlands.

In the distance a group formed by the plane. The women wore yellow-and-brown striped dresses; the men wore the same yellow-and-brown shirts. With them were children from the Lena Ward, some in wheelchairs and on crutches, all moving toward him like a wave. In the middle of these colors he spotted Carin's father in a white-collared shirt with a light blue *shuka* over his left shoulder. And next to him was Carin.

She wore a delicate hat with a round brim and bright white gauze flowing down from it. Her layered skirt floated just above the grass. She was like a shaft of light rising from the wave's white crest.

She and her entourage marched the length of the airstrip. Women waved branches and trilled: *Yi! Yi! Yi!* When they were about fifty feet away, her group moved toward his, dancing and ululating, and then retreated. Then his group did the same. The groups went back and forth, each time growing closer, like two people coming together, uncertain at first, then merging. Carin's father took his daughter's hand and said, "I pass my daughter's hand to yours." Above, great gray clouds moved in like a wild herd, and the sky grew dark.

When it was time for the vows, they stood on the stage and faced each other. Carin promised to "join together and to live for others as well and that we may pass life through our children to live, love, and to offer them justice." Dilan gathered himself for a long moment, and then promised "to join, to be with the essence of the world; and when we give life to our children, to give them a life of love so that they will believe in truth, and goodness and peace, because I think that with you all things are possible."

Then thick pelting drops began to fall. Carin looked at Mama Naman, who said, "Rain on a wedding day is a blessing; it means you'll have many children." Carin looked around, and everyone had grins. She squeezed Dilan's hand in case he was worried that she was worried. It was only rain, so Emmanuel Mighay, the hospital's chief nurse and the wedding's master of ceremonies, continued with the program. Seeing that he was getting wet, Carin found an umbrella and held it over his head. Dilan thought, *Yes, this is why I'm marrying this wonderful woman.* Then the thunder and lightning arrived like a late guest. In seconds the tent sagged. Some men poked sagging spots with their herding staffs, and water poured off the edges in waterfalls.

A gust blew Carin's umbrella upward so it looked like an acacia tree. Men drew machetes to cut holes in the brown canvas to let the water through. More gusts, and the tent gave way. A beam smacked a friend of Carin's family in the forehead. Carin's six-foot-seven brother, Maarten, tried to hold up the broken beams. Dilan and Carin helped lift people up who had fallen. Carin's dress was rusty red below her knees and rain-soaked white above. She ran about in her bare feet. Dilan's white shirt became translucent. He loved this: it was like being in an operating room, acting versus observing, helping others get to safety. And besides, what could be better than a storm to remind you that any rich life has them, and that they leave the world greener after they've passed?

Carin found Dilan by the Land Rover, which was piled high with people. They would move the party to the hospital, where it would continue late into the night. Dilan had a boyish grin, like a toddler playing in a puddle.

"Hello, my beautiful wife. Are you all right?"

He wiped a few wet wisps of hair off her beaming face.

"I couldn't be better."

CHAPTER 39

Dilan left Haydom first, back to the States and his new job in South Carolina. He was in love and more optimistic than ever about his teach-first program. Haydom was proof that it worked. Mayegga was headed to medical school, and despite Dilan's earlier reservations, Emanuel Nuwas had grown into a first-rate surgeon. A buzzing fly had helped convince him of that.

He and Nuwas had been in the operating theater doing a procedure on a tall Maasai woman with elaborate henna tattoos. She'd been having headaches for years, but no one had been able to help. Finally she made the long trek over the Mbulu Highlands to Haydom. Her CT scan revealed a massive meningioma, a type of tumor.

Just before the operation, he and Nuwas realized they had no retractors. Dilan quickly bought an aluminum pan in a shop outside the gates and had the ambulance mechanics cut retractor blades. They began the operation, but the Gigli saw snapped, and Nuwas ended up using half of the saw. Nuwas managed to cut a bone flap, and the retractor blades worked just fine, but then a fly flew into the room. It circled their heads as Nuwas removed the tumor. As he finished his final resection, the fly landed on the woman's brain. Dilan waved it off, and it landed on his left hand. Then it jumped to Nuwas's hand.

"This is bad," Dilan said. "Now we're all contaminated. What should we do?"

"We kill the fly and rinse the wound thoroughly," Nuwas said.

Yes, what else could you do? Nuwas had the poise good surgeons need in stressful situations. Even more than his growing surgical competence, Nuwas had the skills of a teacher. When he spoke at *Sala*, people paid extra attention. He took his time to explain things to other clinical officers. He handled problems delicately and with compassion: If he found a storage room in disarray, he complimented the clerk first instead of berating him. When he saw the clerk's smile, he suggested ways to improve the room, gently in a Tanzanian way so that the clerk soon offered his own ideas, made the project his own mission. That was leadership, Dilan thought. That was the kind of person who could transfer what he knew to other Tanzanians. Train the trainers. A few days later, the Maasai woman walked out of the hospital on her own, cured and unaffected by the fly.

He had another reason to be optimistic: more people were talking about the shortage of doctors and surgeons.

This was due in large part to Haile Debas and his estimate that 11 percent of the world's burden of diseases could be averted with surgery. The 11 percent estimate, though crude, sounded an alarm: Vast numbers of people were dying and suffering because of this shortage. The number hinted at a solution—more surgeons. All of this motivated others to do their own research.

In 2008 a Harvard team thought studying the availability of pulse oximeters might be revealing. Hospitals without these simple fingertip oxygen monitors couldn't properly do surgeries. Why not find out how many hospitals had these devices? Do that, and you'd have another way of measuring the surgical deficit.

After poring through data on pulse oximeter availability in ninety-two countries, they came up with another powerful number: an estimated two billion people worldwide didn't have access to surgical treatment.

One of the study's authors was Atul Gawande, the best-selling medical writer and associate professor of surgery at Harvard Medical School. Later at a medical conference in Boston, Gawande joined Paul Farmer and other prominent global health leaders in a discussion about the world's surgery gap. Gawande told a story about a patient he met in India who could barely breathe. The man had been to one hospital and clinic after another but received minimal treatment. X-rays revealed a tubercular abscess. His lungs were full of fluid. But the hospital didn't have a chest tube, so Gawande and a local doctor wrote a prescription and sent the man's brother to a medical supplier. The brother returned with the tube, but then Gawande and the local doctor discovered that the operating room didn't have any knives. The brother was sent to buy more supplies. By the time he returned, his brother was dead.

"Surgery is an indivisible, indispensable part of health care, but it is treated as a luxury," Gawande would later write.

Also in 2008 another Harvard-led team came up with the first ever estimate of the total number of surgeries done every year across the world—a staggering 234 million operations.

The research team then examined where these procedures were done. They discovered that the richest third of the world's population accounted for 75 percent of the surgical procedures while the poorest third made up just 4 percent. The conclusion was unmistakable: in many places, surgery was the province of the wealthy.

Citing Haile Debas and his colleagues, Paul Farmer and Jim Kim, cofounders of Partners in Health, pleaded for the world to wake up. They knew firsthand about the surgical crisis from their work in Haiti. Over time their clinics had become the country's surgery provider of last resort. In March 2008, the same month that Dilan and Carin were married on the airstrip, Farmer and Kim wrote in the *World Journal of Surgery*, "Although disease treatable by surgery remains a ranking killer of the world's poor, major financers of public health have shown that they do not regard surgical disease as a priority, even though, for example more than 500,000 women die each year in childbirth; these deaths are largely attributable to an absence of surgical services."

Farmer and Kim urged hospitals in wealthy countries to "twin" with ones in poor countries. Surgical supplies should be donated; short-term medical missions needed to be scrutinized for their pros and cons but not abandoned altogether; they called for more money. A huge infrastructure had grown up around infectious diseases, including the Global Fund to Fight AIDS, Tuberculosis, and Malaria. "But there is no Global Fund for Surgery, and rare indeed are the foundations willing to support surgery as an important part of global public health." Surgery, they said, was "the neglected stepchild of global health."

As more researchers discovered the seriousness of the surgical deficit, others raised new questions about traditional humanitarian practices and models. In one study, two Duke University researchers examined inventory reports at hospitals in sixteen countries on four continents. Their goal was to better understand what happened to medical equipment after it was donated.

In all, they looked at the operational performance of more than 112,000 donated machines. They found that nearly 40 percent were out of service. And they uncovered one reason why: North American hospitals typically had service contracts to maintain these delicate pieces of machinery, but service contracts rarely followed the donated equipment overseas. As a result, the authors concluded, hospitals ended up with "an inoperative piece of equipment and a disposal problem."

Later, a group of researchers from the United States and India began a massive study comparing short-term medical missions with other surgical delivery platforms, such as Mercy Ships, and specialty hospitals dedicated to specific procedures, such as the Aravind Eye Hospitals in India.

They soon found a pattern: Short-term missions to treat simple procedures, such as tonsillectomies, generally were safe. But surgical missions that did more complex operations had significantly higher mortality and complication rates. Among their findings: Death rates from hernia operations by short-term teams were twenty times higher than in high-income countries. Meanwhile, the specialty hospitals did more procedures and with fewer complications. The authors concluded that short-term surgical missions should be "limited to areas and conditions for which no other surgical delivery platform is available."

In love and thrilled with what was happening in Haydom and beyond, Dilan headed to South Carolina with a sense of overflowing possibilities. Except for one part of his life: his NGO was struggling. Doctors from Harvard, Duke, the University of Colorado, and other universities were signing up to do teaching missions. Yet, overall, Physician Training Partnership was still a minor player, and the group's trajectory wasn't promising.

Robert Hamilton and some of the volunteers had bickered over the program's lack of direction. Now he and Hamilton were on opposite coasts. His mother still helped with the books; operating costs mainly went on his credit cards. He had made progress while he was in Tanzania, but in the back of his mind he wondered, *Will the NGO and its ideas gather force or peter out?*

Carin stayed a month longer; there was so much to do in Lena Ward.

The ward had been running smoothly before the honeymoon, such a change. When she'd begun, many nurses and students seemed resigned to failure; they came to work unmotivated and glum. But over the months the halls brightened with laughter and higher notes of people enjoying their jobs. With better diagnoses, more children survived instead of ending up on the roster of dead in the morning report. Nurses and others from Moshi and other hospitals had visited Haydom to learn about its success. Nurse Angela had been reluctant at first to get close to Carin. After a few months, they laughed so hard they had to hold each other up.

But in her absence, Lena Ward moved backward. While she and Dilan vacationed mortality rates increased. As they relaxed and camped, children died from missed diagnoses of pneumonia and asthma. When they returned she found that once again too many boys and girls were on antimalarial medicine when they had meningitis. The guilt and loss were overwhelming at times; she felt the ward's regression deep in her gut, as if she'd lost an unborn child.

She believed in Dilan's ideas about teaching, and she had done it here and there with the nurses and clinical officers, but she hadn't done what Dilan had done with Mayegga and Nuwas: find someone to replace her.

It didn't make sense. *I was teaching them like crazy, but it didn't stick,* she told herself. Emma, her colleague from the Netherlands, also had tried to teach and failed. And yet, Dilan's teaching had taken hold. Why had his approach worked?

Then it dawned on her. Yes, she and Emma had done lots of teaching, but their primary focus was still on treating patients. Teaching was secondary, and the staff knew this. But Dilan had made it abundantly clear that he was there only to teach Mayegga and Nuwas. It was a subtle difference in styles, but Dilan's way created a deeper sense of ownership. He taught them brain surgery, but just as important, he taught them to be independent.

Dilan was gone now, and she walked through the wards with a sinking feeling and no appetite. She told herself, *Be more positive.* But her gut wasn't fooled by these affirmations. She realized she was losing weight when her wedding band slipped off more easily. Then one day she realized her finger was bare.

Frantic, she looked everywhere for the ring. It was as if the weight of her decision had caused it to fall off somewhere in Haydom's red soil. During *Sala,* Emmanuel Mighay made an announcement about the missing ring and joked that it didn't really matter because there were so many witnesses at the wedding. Soft and sympathetic laughs rippled through the chapel as Carin raised her eyebrows and shrugged her shoulders as if to say, "I'm sorry for being me."

Then a few mornings afterward, she was on the path from the library to her cottage, her mind pacing through the day's unfinished tasks. Beyond the jacaranda trees and just a few steps away from where Dilan had first seen her, something caught her eye. A sparkle. And there it was, the ring, a tiny mirror glinting in the sun. She placed it back on her finger. It was time to go.

She said good-bye to the Namans, Mayegga, Oystein Olsen, the mechanics. She met Angela in the Lena Ward and saw a distance in her eyes that she hadn't seen for many months. They made small talk, but what she wanted to say was "I'm so sorry."

"Of course you have to go," Angela said, giving Carin a slightly formal hug. Over the years, the staff had learned well how to say good-bye.

PART 3

Teach One

Independence cannot be real if a nation depends upon gifts and loans.

—JULIUS NYERERE,
first president of Tanzania

Years before, when he was in Parliament, Jakaya Kikwete came upon a baffling sight. He and several colleagues were driving to a village near the Usambara Mountains in one of the poorest regions in Tanzania. Average incomes there were less than a dollar a day. Average life expectancies hovered just below fifty years. In the distance, Kikwete spotted four men on the road. They were struggling to balance an enormous basket on a bicycle.

A gregarious man with a ready smile, Jakaya Kikwete had politics in his DNA: his grandfather was chief of a coastal village; his father was a district commissioner in colonial Tanganyika; and on that day riding toward the village, Kikwete was a rising star in the country's dominant political party. His car passed the men and their giant basket, but on the way back he saw them again. They had made little progress. He asked the driver to stop.

He climbed out of the car and looked inside the basket. There, curled in pain, was a pregnant woman. She had been in labor for three days. She was in too much pain to walk to the health center, which was about thirty kilometers away. A basket on a bicycle was her only option.

Kikwete told his driver to take the woman and her family to the clinic; he and his colleagues would wait on the side of the road. As the car drove off, he wondered whether the woman would survive. What about her child? When the driver returned, he told him to take him back to the health center. There, he found the woman had already given birth to a son. She had named him Jakaya.

He would remember that woman's plight through the 1990s when he became foreign minister, and then in the mid-2000s, when he ran for president on the motto "A better life for every Tanzanian. It is possible." Her story showed how poverty and poor access to health care created its own kind of contagion; the woman's difficult labor not only affected mother and child, it also spread to those who tried to wheel her to the clinic. Lack of access to health care added even more unpredictability to their lives. And when you lived at subsistence levels, chance could be the difference between life and death. Would the woman and child be alive now if he hadn't stopped to help them that day?

That moment on the road was revealing in other ways: It demonstrated his people's determination to take care of one another. And it showed how sometimes you need a lift to move forward. In 2005 Jakaya Kikwete was elected Tanzania's fourth president. In 2008, three years into his first term, he was still asking himself, *What can I do to help people like that woman in the basket?*

By that time Tanzania's economy had sprung to life. It had one of Africa's highest economic growth rates. New skyscrapers went up in Dar es Salaam. New cell phone towers bypassed the need for telephone and Internet cables. New banking systems were built based on mobile phones. "The benefit of being late," Jakaya Kikwete sometimes told visitors about these rapid technological advances.

And yet, 42 percent of the government's budget still came from foreign donors. Churches still ran about 40 percent of the hospitals and provided 46 percent of the nation's hospital beds. Tanzania still had some of the world's worst health indicators: 44 percent of children under five had stunted growth because of disease and poor nutrition. Economically, Tanzania was moving quickly from low-income status to middle-income as Jakaya Kikwete had hoped. But like those family members and their basket on the bicycle, the country's health care system was making little progress. What could he do about this?

On September 17, 2008, six months after the wedding on the airstrip, President Jakaya Kikwete traveled to Haydom. He had made health care and education top priorities. Malaria, AIDS, and tuberculosis were killers, but the memory of the woman in the basket reminded him of another troubling problem: his country needed more doctors.

Escorting him through the wards in Haydom were Isaack Malleyeck, an assistant medical officer, and Emmanuel Mighay, the head nurse who had been master of ceremonies at the wedding. In the Lena Ward, Kikwete picked up a baby and spoke about malnutrition. In Radiology, he marveled at the CT scanner from Norway's Friends of Haydom charity—such an advanced piece of machinery in such a remote area!

"The hospital is able to do many kinds of advanced procedures, including brain surgery," Mighay said.

"Brain surgery?" Kikwete asked.

"Yes, we have young guys doing this."

Mighay didn't mention that the guy who did those operations wasn't there anymore—and wasn't so young, either.

CHAPTER 41

A month into medical school Emmanuel Mayegga was ready to quit. His first exam scores were horrible. In a way, he wasn't surprised. Ever since he arrived in Dar es Salaam, he'd found his mind adrift.

Dar could do that to you. It rarely cooled at night as it did in Haydom; the Indian Ocean held the heat and moisture like a hothouse. And the movement and scents inside this hothouse made you dizzy: traders packed Kariakoo's market, filling its stalls with spices, vegetables, and fish; static-soaked loudspeakers issued Muslim prayer calls five times a day; women carried juice pitchers on their heads past shops hawking smartphones; men in red Maasai blankets walked with men and women in business suits. Already packed with four million people, Dar es Salaam was the ninth fastest growing city in the world. Dar was an elephant; Haydom was an ant.

And Mayegga felt out of place in other ways. He was nearly twice as old as some students. He hadn't cracked open textbooks for years. When it came to studying, his neural wiring was rusty. Besides, he was a surgeon. Maybe not officially, but he was used to doing things, not reading about them. Most of all, he thought of those he'd left behind: his wife, Samwayma, and their son, Godwin, growing taller in his absence. He thought about the baby girl they had lost. *Will we have more children? How can you build a family when you are so far away?*

He had enrolled in the International Medical and Technological Institute, one of five medical schools in the country. He'd taken a room in a neighborhood across Old Bagamoyo Road. Long cinder-block fences lined the dirt road to a hill, where trees shaded a row of wooden kiosks. One stall advertised a plumbing service, another sold mangos and sodas. Across from the plumber, a short path led to his room in a building attached to another family's house. Chickens zigzagged past his door, which was protected by a gate made of rebar. Inside, he had a fan and a wooden couch. A picture of a white baby hung high on the wall across from the couch. He wasn't sure where the portrait had come from, and he didn't care; this wasn't home.

Over and over, he phoned Baba Naman. "Why am I here?"

Just keep moving forward, Naman would say. That medical degree will be worth it in the long run. And by the way, another Tanzanian doctor had just arrived in Haydom, Hayte Samo, fresh out of medical school. And Hayte had joined Nuwas in the operating theaters. Keep it up, Naman said, and someday you will be operating again as well.

Baba Naman was right, Mayegga thought. If he continued, he would have more options. Especially if he moved permanently to Dar es Salaam. So many other medical students from rural areas did this. Why not? In a weekend doing private-practice work, you could make enough to send a child in Haydom to school for an entire year. You could become a wealthy person, rich enough to buy a car or a house in one of Dar's suburbs.

But those exam marks! Suddenly the choice seemed clear: he could quit and return to Haydom a failure or push forward as Baba Naman had said.

The next morning, he woke up at 6 a.m. and took the dirt road down to the school. A quick run across Old Bagamoyo Road and he was at the school's three white arches and black metal gate. He hurried to the other end of the campus and a white four-story building with open balconies on each floor. He climbed a stairwell and just above the second floor found a corner that overlooked a threadbare lawn. The floor was painted a shade darker than the red dirt in Haydom. This spot would do. Now and then a hot breeze flowed through the stairwell and the balcony's balusters. He pulled out the textbook, turned the pages. Sometimes you take a step backward to move ahead.

·   ·   ·

In 2009, with Mayegga gone to medical school, Emanuel Nuwas faced his own decision: *Do I operate? Or do I let the patient die?*

With Mayegga and Dr. Dilan, he'd learned enough anatomy to diagnose certain brain diseases, even though he hadn't yet learned how to fix these problems. Such was the case with Charles, an onion farmer who lived in a field below Mount Haydom. A year and a half before, Charles had felt an itch around his eye but thought nothing of it. Then his vision blurred, and then he lost his eyesight altogether. Fearing he had a disease or a curse and would die anyway, his wife and children moved away. His neighbors looked after him for more than a year and then finally took him to the hospital. From his hut it was a fifteen-minute ambulance ride to the gates.

Baba Naman had done the CT scan, which showed a tumor in the frontal lobe. The tumor had damaged nerves to his eyes. Nuwas had never removed a tumor in such a delicate area of the brain. And he had no one to turn to for help.

Mayegga was gone, and Dr. Dilan had left for South Carolina after the wedding. Dr. Dilan had said that other doctors associated with his NGO would soon rotate in and out of Haydom, surgeons from Harvard, the University of Colorado, and the Medical University of South Carolina. But they weren't there now. And besides, could he truly depend on these foreign doctors? Like the brown twisters that popped up in the valley, he had no idea where and when they would show up.

He felt the weight of his decision. If he didn't operate, Charles would be sent home. He could barely move his limbs and would suffer tremendous pain before his final breaths. What message would this suffering send to the community? Would they say the hospital was powerless to help people? Or that the staff just didn't care? No wonder Charles's neighbors had taken so long to bring him here.

Nuwas walked to the hospital's library and piled textbooks and anatomy books on the table. The pages hissed as he turned them. He mapped out the anatomy. He broke the procedure into parts and memorized each step. The more he learned, the more nervous he became. Some blood vessels fed the tumor and others fed the brain. No problem if you cut one to a tumor. But slice through one feeding the brain and Charles would have a stroke.

No one would blame him if he declined to do the operation. After all, he wasn't truly a surgeon. He was just a young doctor out of medical school. He had no formal surgical training—nothing like the surgical residencies that Dr. Dilan and other North American surgeons had gone through. But as soon as he cut the man's flesh, the calculus of responsibility changed. If he failed, people would ask, *What did you do wrong?* Hours passed, and he closed the textbooks.

The theater was a thirty-second walk through the Old Ward and a breezeway. The changing room had wooden cubbies for his pants and shirt. He donned a green cap and green scrubs. A right turn from the changing room led into a dim hallway and the sinks. He scrubbed his hands, and his thick fingers grew soapy. He entered the double door to the theater and scanned the instrument tray. He put on a white gown and rubber gloves. The man lay faceup on the table.

Nuwas picked up a No. 10 scalpel.

Charles didn't die on the table. That had been Nuwas's biggest fear—losing someone with blood and tissue on his surgical gloves.

He checked Charles every chance he had. After a few days, Charles opened his eyes, and then several days after that, he moved his limbs for the first time in months. A week later he walked, and soon he was ready to be discharged. He had saved the man's life but not his eyesight. The tumor had permanently destroyed the nerves. *A shame*, Nuwas thought. Had the man's neighbors brought him in sooner, he might have been able to save those nerves. But at least Charles could go home to his *shamba* farm now. Later, Nuwas learned that Charles's wife never came back, but that several of his children did and had begun to help him around the hut. Wasn't this success?

He'd had other successes throughout 2009: he inserted a VP shunt into a psychotic young man, and the man's erratic behavior all but disappeared; he removed a meningioma the size of an orange from a woman who lived near Mount Hanang, and after she left the hospital, she wrote a letter: "Dear God, thank you for the hands of Dr. Nuwas and the healing that I got from him." Yes, you could do miraculous things with a Gigli saw and forceps.

But, as the months passed, he reminded himself, *I'm not truly a surgeon; I am just a doctor who has learned some surgical procedures.* Dr. Dilan and Mayegga had provided the foundation. But to reach his full potential, he would need specialized surgical training—four more years of school in Dar es Salaam or Moshi.

His thoughts moved to Dr. Dilan and how he'd taught Mayegga, and how Mayegga had then taught him. His mind formed the image of a chain.

He was the end of that chain. If he left, people in Haydom would have nothing to grab. He could hear their voices: *Why is there no one to help me?* People would die in his absence without another link.

Dilan and his NGO doctors couldn't help him forge one. Their appearances were unpredictable. And what's a blacksmith without metal? He would need to find this steel on his own—without the help of any foreign doctors or NGOs.

But who?

What about Hayte?

Hayte Samo had just finished medical school. If he taught Hayte surgery, then Nuwas could leave for surgical training; he could accomplish his own goals, and through Hayte, help those he left behind. He wouldn't have to wait for Dilan's doctors. If he did nothing, though—if he didn't teach someone—then that chain would break. As with his decision to operate on Charles, he had to do something.

But Hayte? Hayte's path to get an MD had been full of zigzags— even moments when he'd stepped off his designated path altogether. Then again, his story was remarkable, even among Haydom's other local doctors. Hayte could teach people a thing or two about persistence and goals.

But could Hayte really do surgery?

Hayte with the fractured spine.

CHAPTER 42

Eight years before, Hayte Samo squeezed into a Mission Aviation Fellowship plane on Haydom's airstrip. Hayte was a handsome man in his twenties with long eyelashes and dark eyes that made him look at once childlike and serious. He smiled with his eyes instead of his cheeks and lips, which added to his serious demeanor. With his sensitive eyes, he gave the impression of someone who had experienced long periods of sadness. On each cheek, he had three downward slashing scars, marking him as Datoga. The plane shook as it rolled down the grass. Soon he would be in Moshi to register for his first year in medical school. Now, perhaps, he would make his father proud.

Then, high over the village of Tumatti, the pilot suddenly shouted into the radio, "No engine!" The pilot emptied the fuel tanks. Hayte felt the plane twist sideways and fall.

Hours later, he was back in Haydom, this time on a hospital gurney. Rescuers had plucked him and the others from the wreckage. Bushes had cushioned the impact so that everyone survived, but the crash left Hayte with a badly broken spine.

He spent months in the hospital. At first, he wondered whether he would stand again, and then as he gained strength, how the crash would affect his plan to become a doctor. He reenrolled a year later, attending classes in a wheelchair, and then as he grew stronger, on crutches. When he told instructors he was interested in surgery, they said, "I'm sorry, you'll never be a surgeon with a spine like that!" But people in his past had said similar things, and he'd always proven them wrong, especially his father.

. . .

His father had five wives who bore thirty-three children, twenty-nine of whom survived. Hayte was the eldest male of the first wife. He wasn't sure when he had been born, only that it was during a year of heavy rain. He was a stubborn boy, perhaps the most mischievous of his father's children, curious about everything he touched, especially the beehives his father kept to make honey for *pombe*, a homemade brew.

When his father harvested the combs, he handed Hayte chunks to lick. Hayte loved honey so much that he demanded more. When his father refused, he decided to make his own. He'd seen bees fly around hives, and he thought of something else that attracted flying insects. He slaughtered a baby goat, tied a rope around its neck, and hung it over a tree branch. Soon, insects buzzed around his special hive; soon, he would have his own honey. Wouldn't his father be proud?

His father beat him with a stick. Later, Hayte took his father's panga machete and used it to make his own *boma*. Instead of thorn branches, he and his playmates cut down an acre of maize and used the stalks. Out came his father's stick again. Another beating came after he watched a veterinarian vaccinate his father's cattle. It gave him an idea for a game: He lined up the other children between two rows of thornbushes and told them to pretend they were cattle. He called them one by one and vaccinated each child with a thorn. Wailing children filled the *boma*.

In desperation, his father decided to send Hayte to school. Many Datoga elders had no use for school because it took children away from herding duties. But his father had heard that teachers punished naughty children. Maybe they could put his son on a better path.

Hayte's school was under two trees, a tall one with a teardrop-shaped canopy for younger children, and one with a wider and shadier canopy across the path for older students. Under the trees, he found answers to how things worked. But much too soon, his father decided that his son's schooling would end. The teacher had done a good job. His son was obedient and respectful. He would be a good shepherd.

But like his hunger for honey, young Hayte loved school too much to accept his father's edict. In the mornings he moved the cattle into the brush and thornbushes and went to school anyway. After school he collected the cattle and brought them home. When his father asked what he had done during the day, he said, "I spent my time with the cattle."

Older boys caught him and beat him for lying. In Hayte's mind, a good day became one in which he went to school and returned home without a beating. Over time his father eventually relented and let him attend school, but only with the understanding that Hayte would quit soon.

But Hayte kept going. He was an excellent student, among the best in his class in primary school, good enough for secondary school if he scored well on a national exam. Which he did. In fact, Hayte earned the top score in the district, which meant he could go to a school near the Ngorongoro Crater, one of the best secondary schools in the region.

Classes were in English, and many students had trouble learning this new language. But he picked it up quickly. After classes he translated what the teacher had taught in English. He did this to survive; his family sent him almost no money. So he taught lessons in exchange for soap; he didn't need to buy books because he used theirs to teach them. His fellow students nicknamed him "Teacher."

Hayte had his sights set on becoming a doctor now, a doctor who did surgery. When it finally came time to graduate, families cheered as their children walked across the stage to accept their academic awards. Hayte earned the top spot in many of his subjects, but each time his name was called the audience was silent. No one had come to see him graduate and cheer for his accomplishments. As far as his family was concerned, it was as if he'd disappeared into the bush. After the ceremony, the father of one of his classmates gave him a hug and asked, "Are you an orphan?"

After the plane crash, Hayte contracted tuberculosis. The bacterium attacked weaknesses in the body, and it went to his fractured discs. He spent hours in bed writhing in pain. His instructors continued to discourage any ideas of becoming a surgeon. By then it was 2007, and he heard that an American neurosurgeon named Dr. Dilan was in Haydom. Perhaps he could offer some advice about his spine.

He traveled to Haydom and found Dr. Dilan, who would soon be married to the Dutch pediatrician, Dr. Carin. Dilan was about to do a craniotomy and a brain tumor resection with Mayegga and Nuwas. After talking with Hayte about his spine, Dr. Dilan had asked, "Do you like surgery?"

"Yes," he said with a serious look.

"Why don't you scrub in?"

In the theater Dr. Dilan turned to Hayte. "Can you tell me the difference between the abnormal part of the brain and the normal part?"

"Yes," he said, and then pointed out the tumor.

"Have you observed Mayegga cut it?"

"Yes," he answered.

"Would you like to try?"

Hayte thought, *Me? I'm just a medical student!*

But then the American gave him a scalpel. He showed him how a brain surgeon held it—like a pencil instead of a butter knife. He handed him forceps and guided his hand toward the patient's brain so he would know the right amount of pressure to use. Until then, he had only cut into cadavers. He touched the patient's brain. He was astonished by its beauty. He felt it pulse with the patient's heart. Smiling with his eyes, he used the forceps to snip off a piece of tumor.

"Very good!" the neurosurgeon had said. "I think you will become a surgeon one day!"

You will become a surgeon one day.

That moment opened something inside his mind. Yes, it might be possible to be a surgeon after all. After his visit with Dilan, Hayte Samo returned to medical school in Dar es Salaam, where one of Tanzania's few surgeons rebuilt his discs with two metal rods, one on each side, fixed with screws. Now with his back rebuilt, he could stand for hours.

He'd cut his own path over the years, and now that path had brought him back to the plateau. *You will become a surgeon one day.* In Haydom Lutheran Hospital, he'd found Emanuel Nuwas eager to teach him surgery. And Nuwas was an excellent instructor. He showed Hayte a procedure, then had him assist with the retractors, and then handed him the scalpels and retractor blades to do the procedure on his own. Soon he was drilling burr holes and inserting VP shunts.

Eight years after the plane crash, he was a doctor learning brain surgery thanks to Dr. Nuwas, and also because no matter who told him something was impossible, he kept moving forward until the impossible happened.

CHAPTER 43

The land around Charleston, South Carolina, is called the Low-country. Twice a day, tides send water miles inland. Because the area is so flat and close to sea level, water and land trade places, usually in marshes of pluff mud and grass. In this soppy place the air is thick with humidity; as it hangs over the marshes the air can feel like just another iteration of water. Unlike a surgeon's blade the Lowcountry is a place of undefined edges.

The Medical University of South Carolina sits on the edge of the Ashley River, and since the campus is so close to sea level, streets in the area fill with saltwater when the moon's tug is strong. At high tide, it percolates up from the storm drains and pools by the curbs.

Like the moon, hospitals generate their own gravity, and MUSC is no exception. It's a dense cluster of older and newer high-rises built of red bricks and sealed windows. MUSC's unremarkable brick buildings hide remarkable machines: gamma knives shoot radiation beams at tumors; lithotripters blast kidney stones with shock waves; helicopters stand ready to scoop up patients in car wrecks. MUSC has eleven thousand doctors, nurses, students, and staff. In a given year, the university generates revenue of $1.7 billion.

In 2009 the population of the Charleston metropolitan area was about 650,000, and about twenty neurosurgeons at MUSC and several other hospitals served these people. Roughly twenty neurosurgeons also practiced in Tanzania and Kenya, with their combined populations of about ninety million. But no matter where they practice, neurosurgeons have their hands full. James Watson, one of the discoverers of DNA, once wrote that the human brain is "the most complex thing we have yet discovered in the universe." And complex things often break.

Strokes are among the most serious and frequent of the brain's potential malfunctions. The origin of the term *stroke* stretches back 2,400 years to Hippocrates. The condition was called apoplexy then and means "struck down by violence." Strokes happen when blood vessels clog with plaque or when an aneurysm bursts. Every year fifteen million people worldwide suffer strokes. Six million people die, and five million are permanently disabled. Stroke is not only the world's second-leading cause of death but also the second most frequent cause of disability after dementia.

Smoking, sugary sodas, and fast foods increase risks of stroke, and South Carolina, with its high rate of obesity and its cultural predilections for fried food and sweet tea, is smack in the middle of what health officials call the stroke belt. The belt is more like a vast blob that stretches roughly from North Carolina to Louisiana, with stroke rates four to eight times greater than areas in the Midwest and Northeast. In 2009, some areas in South Carolina had among the highest stroke rates in the nation. MUSC recruited Dilan largely because of his expertise in aneurysms and strokes.

One morning he found himself staring in disbelief at a woman's CT scan. Most aneurysms are tiny balloons hidden inside the brain's lobes. But the one in this woman's brain rose like a mushroom cloud. It started behind her optic nerve and went through the midline to the top and front of her skull. It was as big as a grapefruit, larger than most tumors Dilan had seen. And instead of the tough malignant cells of a tumor, this was a tissue-thin sac of blood and plaque.

His patient's name was Diana Rodwell. She was in her late sixties and lived with her husband, Leonard, two hours north of Charleston near Myrtle Beach. Leonard had noticed that something wasn't right with Diana for months. She ate more slowly than usual and seemed to get confused during car rides. Guessing that her thyroid was acting up, he took her to the emergency room. A CT scan revealed the monster growing inside her skull.

An ambulance rushed Diana to MUSC. It was a Sunday, and by the time Dilan saw her that afternoon she could barely move her arms and legs. A second CT scan showed the aneurysm had begun to bleed. She wouldn't survive much longer. Perhaps forty neurosurgeons in North America would dare touch such a time bomb.

Dilan memorized the shapes and anatomy of the tumor and tried to imagine how he might fix it—and whether to even try. He could decline, but she would die. If he went ahead, then he assumed some responsibility for her fate. You could talk about risks and options, even ask patients to make the final decisions whether to operate. But if a procedure failed, the patient's loved ones could second-guess such decisions. In their grief they might find a lawyer to reinforce these doubts. The American legal system had created an expectation that bad outcomes equaled bad doctors, which wasn't true in the vast majority of failed operations. The reality was that many diseases, and especially those of the brain, were extraordinarily difficult to manage. A better standard was to expect a doctor to try his or her best, and then when mistakes or bad outcomes happened, learn from them. But that standard could seem inadequate after the loss of a loved one. In a given year, 20 percent of America's neurosurgeons are sued, more than any other medical specialty.

Dilan hadn't been sued, and he wanted to keep it that way. But he also knew what he could do inside someone's brain, so in his mind telling Leonard that it was inoperable was a lie. "If we do this right, she could have close to a full recovery," he said, looking Leonard in the eye. "But I'd say that there's a seventy-five to eighty-five percent chance that we won't get it right."

The alternative was worse—a one hundred percent chance that she would die. Standing there in the ICU, Leonard told him to do the best he could.

In the OR, scrubbed, masked, and gowned, Dilan removed part of her skull. He made an incision on her abdomen and slipped the skull flap into a pocket in the abdominal wall. Doing this would preserve the bone until the swelling in her brain went down. He sliced through her dura and positioned the operating microscope. With his eyes pressed to the lenses, his hands worked quickly to peel apart her hemispheres. Just in time. Fresh blood had clotted under the aneurysm, a sign that it was about to rupture.

"Give me the longest temporary clip you have." A temporary clip would slow blood flow into parts of her brain.

"Give her the thiopental." In small doses, the drug reduces metabolism and the brain's need for oxygen. Larger doses are used to execute prisoners.

"Let me know when five minutes have passed, and then ten minutes."

The race was on; he had twelve minutes to clean the aneurysm sac and set the permanent clip. He cut open the sac. *Shit.* Full of white gunk, plaque, some of it calcified. He sucked out one clot after another, forceps and suckers moving rapid-fire. He set the permanent clip on the aneurysm's neck and removed the temporary clip from the artery.

Done before the circulating nurse said "ten minutes."

A week went by. Residents shook their heads. He knew what they were thinking: *That woman will never wake up.*

But on the tenth day Diana Rodwell opened her eyes. And three weeks later Leonard wheeled her out of the hospital.

As he headed home after cases like this, Dilan felt as if he had finally reached his full potential as a surgeon. He was giving hope to patients who otherwise would die. He made a quick call to Carin to let her know he was on his way and climbed into his truck.

By then, he had traded his old Saab for a 1996 white Ford pickup with a broken air conditioner and saggy seat springs. He sank so low that Carin told him, "It looks as if there's a small child with an enormous head driving your truck."

He climbed into the pickup and followed a four-lane highway over the Ashley River to Folly Road. He let the day's tensions fall away—relaxed that locked-and-loaded look he had at the office. Four lanes turned into two as Folly Road shot across the marsh. As the marsh spread out, he had the same feeling of openness and possibility when he gazed at the plateau toward Hanang. The road ended on a barrier island called Folly Beach.

Folly Beach residents nicknamed their island "the Edge of America," and only partly because of its geography. Some of its residents lived on the fringes as well. On any given day you might see a guy walking down a road in a pirate suit or surfers hanging off a Jeep before they bobbed off a beach known as the Washout.

Their house was perched high on stilts not far from the Washout. From their back porch the marsh grass spread out flat and green. A narrow wooden dock cut through the mud and grass to Folly Creek. With the sun setting, Dilan sometimes watched Carin walk down the center of their long dock: her long arms and legs swinging, her bare feet on the weathered wood planks, her hair scattering, everything moving in a hundred graceful ways. She would stop at the end of the dock and then dive into the creek. She would swim against the current for a while, turn, and follow the current back. When she climbed back onto the dock, her pale skin was a bit flushed, her wet hair slick, and he'd think, *She's the most beautiful person I've ever seen.*

Sometimes, if he made it home early, he dove in with her when the sun was low and the marsh had a yellow-green afterglow. He floated with her, on his back, arms thrown back for balance, supported by the brine. Now and then dolphins appeared, announced by gentle bursts from their blowholes. Then the sun would set, and the crickets would sing, and they would see water bugs skip across the water, tiny white lines of movement, and then the sky would light up with pinks and reds. Folly's sunsets were often more beautiful after the sun went below the horizon.

"Thank you for coming back for me," she would say, recalling how he'd returned to Haydom that November.

"Thank you for marrying me," he would say.

Floating there, he also knew that her mind often drifted back to Haydom. Carin had thought about becoming a pediatrician in the United States, but this meant redoing her residency in an American hospital. That seemed wrong to her, given her high level of training in the Netherlands. They talked about spending more time in Africa someday. But Dilan's work at MUSC was all-consuming; they had just begun to pay down their student debts, and now they had this beach house and a mortgage as high as the house's stilts. So for the next few years they would stay in the States and visit Tanzania when they could.

In the late afternoon clouds built inland and then moved toward Folly Beach and the sea. At the same time the ocean breeze pushed the clouds back. Some days the sea breeze won this tug-of-war and Folly Beach stayed dry. Other times the thunderclouds pushed through. Then the humidity from the marshes and rivers merged with the sky, and it rained as hard as it did during their wedding. Home early from work one humid evening, Dilan climbed the wooden steps of the stilt house, fourteen feet above the sand. He went through the screen door to the porch and then inside. Carin was in the kitchen. She turned, and he saw the tears.

He walked over and wrapped his arms around her. He said nothing, just held her. Ten minutes passed without any words. Then he led her by the hand to a seat in the sunroom. He said almost nothing for another half hour, just kept her close. And then it tumbled out like one of those afternoon thunderstorms. Yes, she was so very happy with their love, and yes, she had abandoned the children in Haydom, and yes, she had worked herself to the edge of exhaustion in Haydom—she could have never sustained that pace—but the sense of purpose she had there was so strong; she had never felt so alive, and yes, she would marry him over and over again, and she would get through these feelings somehow; it's just that she was a missionary doctor—and now her mission wasn't clear.

Holding her tightly, he said, "I only want the true you."

CHAPTER 44

Carin was adrift, and so was Physician Training Partnership. Neural pathways, if not activated over time, eventually disappear like an old country road bypassed by a highway. With his new wife and job, Dilan had let the nonprofit atrophy. He had hoped the force of his ideas would generate enough light to guide others. They would make their own travel plans, build their own relationships with hospitals in East Africa, take over while he and Carin built new lives in South Carolina.

But during his last two visits to Tanzania, student volunteers had argued over their places on buses to Arusha. Dilan snapped at a volunteer who didn't show up at a meeting. When she said that someone should have looked for her, he fired another round: "Our job isn't to look for you." He found himself irked by a volunteer who went to Zanzibar before doing her work in Haydom, even though she was doing it on her free time, and, hell, he had gone to Zanzibar himself to relax. Several volunteers left the group altogether, and others waited for more direction. Because of his many clinical and teaching duties at MUSC, they never heard from him.

Robert Hamilton and others had long struggled with Dilan's tendency to procrastinate. Dilan had been difficult to reach in Portland but was even harder to pin down now. Then when you had him on the phone, he might second-guess work you spent months on. It was a classic case of "founder's syndrome." Conversations stopped when Dilan walked into a room; people signed up immediately to work with his NGO after they heard him speak; everyone was energized by the creativity he unleashed. But Hamilton had a nonprofit to run, and all the rules, logistics, and administrative details that came with one. Dilan seemed to regard these rules as impediments to the creative process. Over time Hamilton grew tired of playing the bad cop. Later, Hamilton began a consulting relationship with the Barrow Neurological Institute in Arizona. By then Dilan felt as if his director was working for other groups, not his. They parted ways near the end of 2008. His nonprofit had been on life support since then.

"This is terrible," he told Carin one night. "Tanzania is ready for us, but our organization here in the States is a train wreck."

Dilan and Carin met D and Jane Word at a neighborhood party on a dock that overlooked Folly Creek. Carin and Jane clicked like the nail gun that Jane sometimes carried around at home. "Chick with a gun," Jane occasionally warned her husband. Jane was an artist with swirls of auburn hair; she worked with fiberglass and wore tropical green pumps. A twelve-foot fiberglass lizard was attached to the chimney of their home. Neighbors sometimes knocked on the door of "the Lizard House" to see her latest incarnation: a toilet seat shaped and colored green like a lily pad; curtain rods formed like live oak branches. D Word was delighted. "Darling," he would say in his big northern Alabama twang, "this is our forever house, so do whatever you'd like, because I know it will be beautiful."

D Word preferred that people just call him D because he never thought his given name, Doyle, fit—and he was right. He was six-foot-three, with curly hair and a voice as expansive as his build. He was an Air Force veteran of Vietnam who went into textiles. He'd run Canadian Uniform Limited, a textile company in Ontario, and, in 2009, was just about to retire as chief executive officer of Steiner Systems, a hygiene product maker in Chicago. The last thing Carin and Dilan expected to hear about this bear of a man was his pioneering role in pantyhose.

D would explain: Earlier in his career, a customer from Miami made pantyhose for oversized women, but Hanes and other big players had muscled into his market. D Word's company was selling gussets that went into tights, and after thinking about it, he said, "How about a cotton crotch?" The customer thought he was joking, but D, who had an engineering degree, said that moisture evaporates well from cotton pads and might reduce bacteria. The idea took off and eventually became an industry standard.

As he learned about D Word's background, Dilan thought, *Here's an original thinker.* And also: *Here's someone who has extensive international business experience and the managerial skills I lack.* D didn't seem like the kind who would play much golf when he retired. Dilan asked if he would help run his nonprofit.

D wasn't interested. When it came to poverty and disease, he'd long thought that Africa was a lost cause. When the subject of foreign aid came up, D Word would say, "They're just pissing money away."

Dilan pressed: Teaching could break the cycle of dependency; his nonprofit's goal was to teach and then get out.

Teach and leave. "An exit strategy. I like that," D said. He finally agreed to be the director, with one stipulation: His salary would be one dollar.

Soon after, they gathered one night in the Lizard House. Jane had embedded an aquarium in the middle of the kitchen island. A container of hummus sat above the tropical fish. Jane wore a yoga outfit and her fingers sported green nail polish. D Word was in shorts and a shirt as colorful as the fish. The name of the nonprofit came up: Physician Training Partnership.

"I don't want to hurt anybody's feelings, but we need to change that," Jane said.

"But we don't want something that sounds evangelical," added D, who was an atheist. He refilled everyone's wine glasses.

They tossed around names.

"Isn't there anything in Swahili?" Jane said. "What's Swahili for *doctor?*"

"*Daktari,*" Carin said. "The plural form is *madaktari.*"

"*Madaktari, madaktari,*" Jane said, turning it over in different vocal tones.

"I like that," D Word said, growing more excited because Jane was excited.

Grinning, Carin said, "How about Madaktari Africa?"

.   .   .

Madaktari Africa it was. By early 2009, a year after the wedding on the airstrip, Dilan's nonprofit had a new name and a new director. Now they could rebuild the organization and tackle new goals, get it done. Dilan's latest goal wouldn't be easy: build a consensus among his peers in neurosurgery that the overriding purpose of future medical missions should be to teach—a challenge to the short-term missionary model. He imagined the impact: if the neurosurgery establishment took a stand, then that would send a message to the larger medical community that the status quo wasn't working.

His plan was simple and bold. They would get some of the world's most prominent neurosurgeons together in a room in St. Louis. Then he would tell them what they had been doing all these years was quite possibly doing more harm than good.

CHAPTER 45

Three miles west of the Gateway Arch, the St. Louis Medical Society Building stands as a proper edifice to medicine, even though it once housed the National Museum of Quackery. The brick building was built in the mid-1920s and had three white ionic columns at the entrance. The quackery museum, before it moved to another city, had the Orgone Energy Accumulator—a conical cap and a shawl for patients to increase their "cosmic energy"—and a colored light that supposedly cured baldness. Now the building was known worldwide for its practical anatomy and surgical workshops.

On March 4, 2009, neurosurgeons from four continents climbed the building's granite steps. Inside, they passed doors to the anatomy lab where surgeons and students practiced on cadaver specimens. They took a staircase to the second-floor conference room, where they found Dilan and D Word with mugs of coffee. It had been surprisingly easy to bring this group together, partly because some were trying to establish global health programs, but also because of Paul Young.

Young stood about six-foot-two and had unusually steady blue eyes. He'd bought the entire building to create an anatomy lab, which he'd modeled on fantasy baseball camps. Professional teams held such camps so fans could live their childhood dreams of playing in a Major League Baseball stadium with famous ballplayers and coaches. But instead of pitchers and shortstops, Young recruited instructors such as Gazi Yasargil of Turkey, perhaps the most respected living neurosurgeon. With the lab established, Young's steady eyes had focused on global health. He'd been an ally of Dilan's ever since Dilan asked his advice about his work with Mayegga. After Dilan smoothed things over with Moody Qureshi and Abedi Kinasha, Young and Dilan worked together on several East African training projects. Young concentrated on his own program in Kenya, while Dilan worked in Tanzania.

Light poured through tall windows. Moody Qureshi and Abedi Kinasha entered along with Jose Piquer Belloch, head of Spain's top neurosurgical association, and Knut Wester, a Norwegian who had studied ski jump injuries and worked in Ethiopia. Merwyn Bagan, the head of FIENS, arrived, as well as Dilan's mentor at Harvard, Arthur Day. A large group from the Barrow Neurological Institute was there, and among them was Robert Hamilton. With Hamilton was Tom Bible, the son of a wealthy British family who had an aneurysm repaired at the Barrow. Doctors from Cornell, Duke, the University of Colorado, and other leading medical institutions took seats around a wooden table, nine feet wide and twenty-one feet long. It was so large that it seemed to float in the middle of the room. Together this group easily had one thousand academic papers and textbook chapters on their CVs.

Paul Young began by asking everyone for fifteen-minute synopses of their medical mission work, a smart move, Dilan thought. In a room full of healthy egos, you better make sure everyone gets a say. As they spoke over the next three hours, Dilan had two thoughts: *Man, these people have done amazing work.* And, *It's obvious that missions have failed to cure the overall problem.*

When it was his turn, he faced the screen. His first slide was an African proverb: "If you want to go fast, go alone: if you want to go far, go together." Quickly he flashed through photos of Maasai men walking with staffs and his green Land Rover churning through knee-deep mud—he'd snapped them during his honeymoon.

He began, "So what happens to neurosurgical patients in rural Tanzania? Most people die or live with a profound disability. We've addressed this problem with traditional medical missions. We go for a few weeks or maybe a month, and this is great for patients lucky enough to get the operation. It's a wonderful humanitarian endeavor. But it perpetuates a cycle of dependency. We need to solve this problem quickly, because every day this situation persists, people die. Needlessly."

He described his intensive clinical teaching approach with Mayegga and then made his pitch: Let's bring the world's most prestigious neurosurgery organizations, hospitals, and universities under one umbrella and shift our overseas endeavors toward teaching instead of treating. Madaktari Africa could serve as that umbrella and lay the legal and organizational groundwork with East African governments, universities, and other partners.

"But above all, we need to teach. And then teach people how to teach. And how will we know when we're successful?" A silent moment passed. "Success is when we're no longer needed."

Dilan took a seat. Paul Young suggested they discuss what they'd heard. Dilan thought to himself, *This is where it could all fall apart.*

A neurosurgeon from Wisconsin launched into an extended speech about his mission work. Paul Young interrupted, "I'd love to let you have the microphone all day, but this isn't about your work; it's about working on something greater than any one of us." *Another smart move,* Dilan thought. *Focus on a higher goal.*

Tom Bible spoke up about the Barrow's good deeds. Young reined him in more gently. Patients whose death sentences were commuted by a surgeon's hands often had deep emotional attachments to their doctors and hospitals. You had to respect that bond.

Several other neurosurgeons said they were concerned about maintaining control over their programs if they collaborated. It was Dilan's turn to intervene.

"No, keep doing what you're doing." Madaktari Africa would sort out liability, legal, customs, and other technical issues. Let each university and hospital do its own innovative work and take credit for any successes. This was about making it more efficient for everyone and changing the mission paradigm away from treating to teaching.

Paul Young pulled out a paper and pen. "Let's move forward with concrete steps. Here is what I'm hearing: We should come together under an umbrella organization, but we'd have our own nonprofits."

Yes, the neurosurgeons said.

"Madaktari Africa will act as a facilitator."

Yes.

"Do we all agree that the goal of the programs is to teach?"

Agreed.

Done with their work, the surgeons reconvened that night inside a mansion owned by the chairman of St. Louis University's neurosurgery program. The dining room was filled with Persian rugs and fine antiques. The lighting was warm, different shades of orange and brown. The dinner was catered, and the wine flowed. Knut Wester, the Norwegian, jumped onto a chair, did a jig, and sang a folk tune. Dilan took a minute to look around and listen; he heard easy conversations, laughter, the kind of satisfaction you hear in the OR when closing and everyone knows a badly injured patient will be OK.

Euphoric, they left St. Louis determined to build on this momentum.

With D Word and Abedi Kinasha, Dilan traveled to Chicago for a board meeting of FIENS. Because of the groundwork in St. Louis, members of FIENS embraced Madaktari Africa's teach-first approach and created a new East African training program.

In the coming weeks, Dilan and D Word also met with members of the Congress of Neurological Surgeons, who agreed to steer the group's outreach work toward a teach-first model.

Back in Charleston, Dilan approached MUSC's dean with the idea of establishing a global health center. At the time MUSC didn't have an international health program. "Here's our chance to be on the cutting edge of global health," he said. "No other program in the country has as its core principle the goal to teach medical skills to others, and then teach them to teach." He figured it might take five years to get a program up and running. Instead it took four months.

But as the months passed, he and D Word had yet to reach one of their most important goals: a formal partnership with a government in East Africa. They made plans to travel to Tanzania, but then Dilan set them aside for a new priority. Carin was pregnant.

Before she'd left the Netherlands to work in Africa, Carin's doctors said she might never have children. Medicine might help balance her hormones, but there was no guarantee. She'd felt a twinge of disappointment, but her mind was on finishing residency. And then she'd gone to Africa, where that twinge was buried even deeper by the Lena Ward's daily crush of patients. But when she fell in love with Dilan, the disappointment returned, this time in a flood of fear. Would Dilan think less of her and their future together? Gathering her courage, she told him about the diagnosis.

He'd taken a long pause and then looked her in the eye. It didn't matter. "Our love is the foundation. If we have kids, wonderful. That foundation will allow our children to flourish. If we never have children, that will be OK, because we'll still have love."

In South Carolina she was about to see a fertility expert when she discovered she was pregnant. And then in January 2010 she gave birth to Else, who had her mother's long arms and legs and her father's rich brown skin and clamshell ears. Such a gift.

Since leaving Haydom, Carin had experienced bouts of sadness that bled into despair, but these painful periods were also gifts. She had needed to understand what worked in her life and what didn't—why she had wanted to become a missionary doctor, and why in Haydom she had worked herself to the edge of exhaustion.

Over time she'd come to realize that she truly loved the sense of significance and purpose in treating patients. Others, like Dilan, could detach and teach, and she did like teaching, but she needed to do hands-on work. Humanitarian work was often a mix of self-interest and selfless actions. And, there was nothing wrong with this as long as you were honest with yourself. Even better, if you were honest about your motivations, then your heart would open to new possibilities: deeper bonds with the people you helped; a richer understanding of the cultures. You would be less apt to feel like a martyr or have a false sense of superiority.

In choosing love over her dreams of being a missionary doctor, she probably wouldn't become someone like her mentor, Professor Elizabeth Molyneux. Instead, she felt as if she was moving ever closer to her true self. She loved being a wife and now a mother. She thought she would be a doctor again someday, maybe in Africa for part of the year—and as far as that chapter was concerned, she would still take her old mentor's advice and wait. As for the rest, she would delight in what was and what would follow.

CHAPTER 46

That April in Haydom marked the end of a good rainy season. Around the airstrip, *shamba* fields of sunflowers and maize formed a yellow-and-green quilt. It hadn't rained for a few days, and the soil had begun changing from its rainy-season brown to its dry-season ochre. Jacaranda trees inside the hospital's gates flowered and dropped their petals, creating purple blankets over the roots. Set on the red soil, the petal blankets looked like the purple and red *shukas* worn by the Datoga.

In the chapel for *Sala*, Dilan rubbed his eyes and slouched in his chair. He wore a blue long-sleeve shirt with the button-down collar buttons undone. He was groggy from all the flights—eight thousand miles from Folly Beach to Haydom, eight time zones from Carin and baby Else. A bird flew from one rafter to another. The choir began, and soft and rhythmic voices wrapped the room in velvet.

He and Carin had thought about taking this trip together, including Else. But antimalaria medicine would be hard on Else's young body, and malaria itself would be even worse. So they had decided that Carin and Else would stay behind this time. Dilan would go for three weeks—a short-term mission to push Madaktari Africa forward.

After morning prayers, nurses, orderlies, clinical officers, and foreign doctors poured out two double doors. The visitors and the staff formed tributaries to the Lena Ward, outpatient clinic, and operating theaters. Dilan followed one current toward the circular island at the hospital's main entrance. You pass by the circle to reach Radiology, the Old Ward, administration, the canteen, and paths to the guesthouses, so it was the perfect spot to find someone. And he was anxious to see Emanuel Nuwas.

He'd heard that Nuwas was doing extraordinary work. Months before, Sunil Patel, Dilan's immediate supervisor at MUSC, had come to Haydom on his own, partly because he loved to teach but also to find out why Dilan spent so much time here. After all, Patel had a department to run, and when one of his neurosurgeons was in Africa, he and the others had to fill the gap.

Patel observed Nuwas operate and taught Nuwas new procedures, and he returned to South Carolina thinking that Dilan was on to something. You truly could teach neurosurgery in the African bush. And, yes, if you could do it there, you could do it anywhere. He was so enthusiastic that he made plans to fly back to Tanzania. He would join Dilan and D Word later in the week in Dar es Salaam.

Within seconds Dilan spotted Nuwas, who was in his white doctor's coat. Dilan grabbed his hand and brought him in for a hug. Next to Nuwas, Hayte Samo stood patiently, and then Dilan gave him a bear hug as well. Hayte Samo had news: Nuwas had begun to teach him brain surgery.

"I'm being trained by the master," he said. "I can do spina bifida and VP shunts. The credit is to Nuwas."

Dilan beamed. First Mayegga, then Nuwas, and now Hayte.

Nuwas said he had something to show him. Through a side door, they entered the radiology meeting room. Black curtains covered the windows, and the overhead lights were off. Nuwas sat at the computer in the rear of the room and clicked the mouse. The monitor brightened their faces as a CT scan came up.

"When she came in, she did not know what was happening," Nuwas said. "She was semi-conscious. She could not control her urine or bowels, and she was sick for a long time. We did a CT scan and found a big tumor in the frontal lobe. So we operated."

Dilan leaned over Nuwas's left shoulder with Hayte just behind. The tumor was the size of an apple.

Nuwas said he spent four hours in the theater. "Now the patient is at home. She is fine. Her life is renewed."

Dilan stood straight and took a step back from the computer. To reach the tumor, Nuwas navigated fragile blood vessels like a pilot flying through a mountain range. A good number of North American brain surgeons would have passed on such a risky operation.

"Dr. Nuwas, this is as complex a brain surgery as you'll find anywhere in the world." He shook Nuwas's hand, then slapped his shoulder. "I'm telling you, this is what it's about! What you're doing is beautiful! You're the second generation. Mayegga, now you. And Hayte. This will be in the *Journal of Neurosurgery* one day!"

This was huge, he thought. And not just because of what Nuwas had done to the woman's brain. Nuwas had taught Hayte Samo without any prodding from him or Madaktari Africa. *That is true independence*, he told himself.

But forward momentum brings headwinds. As they went through more CT scans, a young radiologist from Belgium appeared at the door. He had short brown hair and bright eyes, and he spoke in excitable bursts. He moved to the computer and took the mouse from Nuwas.

"Look how beautiful it is," he said. "You can tell it's an abscess by these lines."

The Belgian went on, his eyes locked on Dilan's, a familiar pattern. Foreign doctors often made eye contact with him and ignored local doctors standing next to him. He tried to divert their gazes by saying, "He's the neurosurgeon. It's his case." Most of the time, the visiting doctors kept looking at him anyway. Like this earnest Belgian who meant well but had no idea Nuwas had done such an advanced procedure.

As the Belgian continued his lecture, Nuwas fiddled with a pink piece of paper, then did some paperwork. Dilan had a bad feeling.

Confirmation came next morning. He stood in the back of the meeting room as usual. The latest batch of foreign medical students and doctors filed in and crowded into the front seats. He looked around. Except for Baba Naman, no other Tanzanians were present. Fed up, the clinical officers had boycotted the meeting.

The foreign doctors went through the hospital's latest cases. Near the end, Nuwas walked in and took a seat. Dilan raised his voice.

"Guys, look around the room everyone. There's something wrong with this picture. Dr. Nuwas just joined us. But where are the other Tanzanians? None of you will be here a year from now. So that means we are failing our primary job here, and that's to train people."

"That's quite true," a European doctor near the front chimed in.

"But some of the clinical officers don't want our help," a medical student said.

"That's just an excuse," Dilan fired back. "Find out which clinical officers are in your ward, and just grab them. Bring them to Radiology. And make it fun for them. They are the most important people in the hospital."

As the meeting broke, Dilan muttered out loud: "Changing the mind-set—it's a constant battle."

A week later, Dilan and D Word left the crisp air of Haydom for the hothouse of Dar es Salaam. They chartered a Mission Aviation Fellowship plane to fly there directly. After landing they filed through the airport and found a beat-up taxi. The driver immediately drove to a gas station. "That tells you something," D Word said. "The driver can only afford gas when he has a paying passenger."

The streets were packed with trucks, motorcycles, and *dala dala* buses. Young men rode on heaps of garbage in dump trucks. The air carried scents of trash, diesel fuel, and wood smoke. Their route took them into a densely packed district with mosques. Jewelers hawked gold and tanzanite. They stopped in front of the Peacock Hotel, a modern high-rise with bluish-black tinted windows and a lobby with polished marble floors. Near four dark leather chairs they found Sunil Patel talking with a Tanzanian cardiologist named Mohamed Janabi.

Janabi had a manila envelope containing several CT scans. He'd been having terrible headaches and feared he had an aneurysm.

With his youthful face and his dark wire-rim glasses, Mohamed Janabi had a scholarly look about him, as if he'd just graduated from medical school. In fact, he was nearly fifty and was one of Tanzania's most experienced specialists. He had trained in Europe and Asia. In Japan, he received a PhD in cardiovascular disease. He was the personal physician for President Jakaya Kikwete.

Dilan and Sunil Patel took the CTs from the envelope and held them up to the windows. In the CT's shadows and light, they saw some unsettling shapes. They agreed that he should have a CT scan with an angiogram, a test that uses dye to identify blood vessel problems. It was routine in North American hospitals, but as far as they knew, the nearest hospital with the appropriate equipment was in Kenya.

"I'll go with you," Dilan said. If he did have an aneurysm, Janabi would need urgent surgery. No hospital in Tanzania was equipped to do aneurysms. Dilan and Sunil talked it over: If necessary, they would fly him to South Carolina for the operation, and Dilan would do it himself.

Janabi thanked them and hurried out the hotel's sliding glass doors. Several other colleagues from MUSC had also arrived by then, and Dilan joined them in the hotel basement bar. Just after his beer arrived, he heard the bleating tones of his mobile phone. It took a moment to realize who was on the line.

"Please, take care of my physician," the president said.

Dilan pondered the irony after he hung up. Here he was, a neurosurgeon from America, flying to Tanzania to help the country become less dependent on foreign doctors, working now to help the president's doctor fly to Kenya for tests and maybe even surgery in the United States. How was this independence? Was this just another perpetuation of the colonial model? Special preference for an elite doctor?

Dilan returned to his room in the Peacock Hotel and changed into a tan business suit. He had an hour or so before he met Janabi at the airport. He wished he had a bit more time, because there was someone else in the lobby he wanted to see: Emmanuel Mayegga.

He found him there looking relaxed, all smiles, none of the worry lines he'd had on Naman's back patio three years before. He had that old swagger. He wore a white button-down shirt with blue stripes; a pen peeked out of the shirt pocket. He had lots of news!

His wife, Samwayma, had just delivered twins, a boy and a girl. They had lost a child, "but now we are double-blessed." The boy's name was Godlisten, because God had listened to their prayers, and the girl's name was Glory, to give glory to God.

After Dilan shared his news about his new daughter, Else, Dilan's colleagues at MUSC, Kathleen Ellis and Brennan Wesley, asked Mayegga what he thought about Dilan's teach-forward approach.

"My first thought is that I think he is crazy," Mayegga told them. "But he's a man wanting to do something in a place where things are not available. He always wants to do brain tumors and bleeding in the brain and things that we don't do. But we have to do something."

Then he talked about how he'd slept on cattle skins as a child, how he'd been chased by a python, how he'd studied by a kerosene lamp and woken up with soot in his nostrils, and later, how after learning brain surgery, he'd taught Nuwas.

"Yes, I was happy to teach Nuwas because I was on call twenty-four-seven. Now he's doing it himself, and I heard now that he's training Dr. Hayte. That's the whole thing. We can't be jealous of what we have. We have to transfer the knowledge to others."

Dilan sat back in his seat. "It's one thing to teach someone to do something," he told Mayegga. "But it's another to watch someone teach someone else. Fantastic."

The next day in Nairobi, the angiogram completed, Dilan sat with his arm on Janabi's shoulder. A twinkle in his eye, Dilan said, "My friend, I hate to say this, but I will not get the pleasure of operating on your head." The angiogram was normal—no aneurysm. "This is the best news possible, Mohamed."

No one could say for sure what caused the headaches. You can scan the closed box, but its mysteries often remain hidden. Stress could have been a factor. Just as neurosurgeons were in short supply, so were cardiologists. Janabi had been working eighty-hour weeks for months. But the trip to Nairobi was more than worth it: it gave them a chance to get to know one another.

As with many Tanzanians, Janabi was soft-spoken but had steel in his eyes. He had the credentials and experience that could land him a job in any wealthy country. He could easily be one of the thousands of doctors from sub-Saharan Africa who immigrated to North America or Europe. He'd learned advanced procedures in Europe and Asia but only on sophisticated pieces of equipment. In Tanzania, he had none of these machines at his disposal. He couldn't practice medicine to his full potential. He'd grown so frustrated that he nearly decided to move to Europe. But he stayed and now spent a good part of his time trying to improve the country's health care system. He was particularly upset that the government sent employees with severe heart conditions to India and other overseas hospitals. The government paid their overseas hospital bills to the tune of about $7 million a year.

"That makes no sense," Dilan said. "You have no return on your investment. In fact, you are supporting another country's health care system instead of your own."

"That's true, Dylan." Janabi pronounced his name like the American musician Bob Dylan.

Dilan didn't correct him. "So, let's do the training here. We could spend that money on a new heart clinic and teach Tanzanians to do the procedures. They could treat those government employees and anyone else in Tanzania. And once they're trained, they could train a new generation of Tanzanian specialists in other parts of the country."

"Let me work on this," Janabi had said when they returned to Dar.

A few hours later Janabi phoned and asked Dilan to put together a summary of his ideas. "I think you need to meet with the president."

CHAPTER 47

From a distance, the Tanzanian State House looks like an Arabic fortress. It has bright white walls and crenellated towers. The Germans built it before World War I, and the British rebuilt it after it was damaged in the war. The president's private residence was behind it in a contemporary building with cathedral ceilings. Dilan and D Word heard the peacocks calling in the gardens as the guards frisked them.

They were shown to the living room, where Mohamed Janabi stood by two white couches. Next to the couches was a leather chair with a zebra-skin seat cushion. They heard voices of children from a balcony above the living room. Kikwete had eight sons and daughters, and D Word saw a few of them peek through the balcony railing to see who was below.

Moments later Jakaya Kikwete appeared on the balcony steps with the report in his hands. "I was reading this last night. Very interesting."

He wore a casual gray suit over an open-collar black shirt with curving white stripes. He was about a head shorter than Dilan and D Word and looked younger than his age. He would turn sixty that year, but his cigar-brown skin was smooth. Kikwete sat in the zebra-skin chair, leaned back, and crossed his legs. Dilan and D Word sat together on the couch, leaning forward, their feet flat on the floor, as if they might suddenly stand at attention.

D Word, the former CEO, knew that executives like to get to the point, especially after business hours, so he summarized Madaktari Africa's goals and made his pitch: "We're offering you doctors from some of the world's top medical schools to come and teach, basically for free. And when they've trained your people forward, they'll leave. They're not missionaries."

"We need to do something about health care in my country," Kikwete said. "People should get the care that they need."

"It's possible," Dilan said, but it could only happen with a cadre of skilled local health-care workers. He brought up the government's $7 million expense to send heart patients overseas.

"We could equip a clinic and bring a cardiac surgeon and nurses here for a quarter of that cost," he said, purposely using the word *we*. The cardiac surgeon and nurses could then train local doctors and nurses. "We're an independent country. But we're not truly independent as long as we have Westerners like me do the work instead of Tanzanians. Until this paradigm changes, we're still as dependent as we were during the colonial period."

"Yes, that is true," Kikwete said.

Dilan mentioned Haydom, and how he'd taught brain surgery there to an assistant medical officer. "If you can teach brain surgery in Haydom, you can do it with any specialty. And you can do it anywhere."

"An AMO is doing neurosurgery in Haydom?" he asked, Dilan's words jogging a memory. He had been to Haydom; he had seen the CT machine, but he hadn't met any brain surgeons there. "Is this really being done?"

"Yes," Dilan said.

"Oh," Kikwete said. He put his hands on his knees. "That is wonderful."

CHAPTER 48

No one is sure how the brain processes perceptions of time, but the amygdalae often feature prominently in theories. The amygdalae light up in a neural glow when you experience something unexpected; details become clearer; time slows, as it did when Dilan stepped off the tarmac in 2006, his mind processing the wood smoke and starlit Tanzanian sky. And it slowed again that night in 2010, when he and D Word sat down with President Jakaya Kikwete. Dilan would never forget the quality of the presidential china. D Word remembered the dish of cashews.

Neuroscientists also know that our perceptions of time change when we have more things to do than we can reasonably accomplish. Time speeds up under such a crush. And after the meeting with President Kikwete, time gathered speed for Dilan as Madaktari Africa joined the increasingly swift currents of global health.

After the meeting, Mohamed Janabi joined Madaktari Africa as its Tanzanian director. Thanks to Janabi, Dilan and D Word had instant access to the country's top health leaders. In short order, Madaktari Africa signed an agreement with the government formalizing its role as facilitator of teach-first programs throughout the country. D Word insisted on inserting the words *exit strategy* in one of the agreement's conditions.

Back in the States, Dilan and D Word worked with Tanzanian officials and doctors at MUSC to build a heart catheter lab in Dar es Salaam and teach local nurses and doctors to operate it. Finally Janabi and other local cardiologists had the equipment and skilled staff to properly do their jobs. In Mbeya, a city near the borders of Malawi and Zambia, a hospital had received a donation of dialysis machines.

But no one knew how to operate them, and they gathered dust for month after month. Under Madaktari's umbrella, MUSC doctors and staff trained three doctors who taught others. In Mwanza, a city by Lake Victoria, Madaktari Africa worked with the Canadian Network for International Surgery, Cornell University, and other groups to teach neurosurgery and anesthesiology at Bugando Medical Centre.

For years Madaktari Africa was funded out of Dilan's pocket and the pockets of volunteers. Then in 2011, the group landed an $850,000 multiyear grant from the Henry M. Jackson Foundation for the Advancement of Military Medicine. The grant paid for doctors from Baylor University, MUSC, and the University of South Carolina Medical School to teach family medicine, nephrology, and cardiology in Mbeya. By 2011 more than five hundred volunteer doctors and medical students had traveled to Tanzania under Madaktari Africa's banner.

Still, Dilan sometimes found himself imagining what he could do if his nonprofit had more resources. With more money and staff, you could send doctors to Tanzania for longer periods. That investment of time would allow these master teachers to create stronger bonds with local doctors and, as partners, establish truly local training programs. Then other residents and attending doctors could visit for shorter periods to supplement the work of the full-time doctors. The emphasis would always be on intensive bedside clinical instruction. Put them in the fire early. With this boot-camp approach, it wouldn't take long to train a new cadre of Tanzanian surgeons capable of doing basic surgical procedures—a few years perhaps.

Such ideas came amid a growing backlash against short-term missions, particularly in religious circles. "We fly off on mission trips to poverty-stricken villages, hearts full of pity and suitcases bulging with giveaway goods, trips that one Nicaraguan leader describes as effective only in 'turning my people into beggars,'" American minister Robert D. Lupton wrote in *Toxic Charity*. He and other critics were quick to cite waste and blunders: in Liberia, visitors built a school that couldn't withstand monsoons and collapsed, killing two children; in Mexico, missions painted the same church six times in one summer.

And more voices were calling for new train-first programs. Although the word *sustainable* was often overused, many humanitarian groups and campaigns had truly shifted toward a different way of helping the poor. In 2010, for instance, the American Academy of Pediatrics and a large group of NGOs launched Helping Babies Breathe, a program to teach nurses and clinicians how to resuscitate newborns. The campaign taught simple techniques such as keeping newborns warm, massaging them to improve circulation, and suctioning their mouths. The method didn't require new equipment or pharmaceuticals. It was all about skills and mastery—and an important goal was to train "master trainers" to pass these techniques on to others. Haydom Lutheran Hospital and seven other hospitals in Tanzania were part of the campaign's pilot study, and the results were remarkable. Teaching these simple techniques reduced early neonatal deaths by nearly half. During the next three years, the Helping Babies Breathe technique was introduced in more than sixty countries. More than one hundred thousand birth attendants were trained.

Other train-first programs had gathered steam. Smile Train, an early adopter of a train-forward model, flooded mailboxes with photos of deformed children's faces. Its campaigns raised questions about "poverty porn" and how such images reinforced stereotypes about poverty in low-income countries. But the appeals were effective. By 2010 Smile Train was raising nearly $100 million a year. By then, the group had provided free training to sixty thousand medical professionals in more than 140 countries.

Perhaps the most holistic and ambitious train-forward experiment was in Rwanda, led in large part by Paul Farmer and Partners in Health. After the genocidal horrors in the mid-1990s, many had written off Rwanda's health care system. But Partners in Health had been in Rwanda for a decade and forged strong relationships with the country's autocratic president, Paul Kagame, and local health officials. Building on these partnerships, in 2012 the Rwandan government and twenty-five American medical schools and hospital systems launched the Human Resources for Health Program, a model that Farmer hoped would serve as an alternative to traditional short-term medical missions.

All told, the program would deploy about one hundred doctors and other teachers across the country. The group would address brain drain by stocking clinics with new equipment. It would educate a new generation of health care managers; without good hospital management, even the best doctors couldn't do their jobs, a situation that would soon haunt Haydom Lutheran Hospital.

An all-star cast of American medical institutions came together, including Harvard, Yale, Duke, and Columbia. The consortium's goal was to train five hundred doctors in various specialties, including surgery, and increase the skill levels of five thousand nurses. After seven years, the Rwandan government would take over. Farmer didn't like the term *exit strategy*. At the end of the funding cycle, the group hoped that doctors in both countries would have strong enough bonds to continue collaborating but as equal partners. In the first year, the consortium did more than six hundred lectures and seventy thousand hours of bedside teaching. Life expectancy and other health indicators were rising.

Part of its success involved money—the program had a seven-year budget of $150 million. Funds came from the Global Fund to Fight AIDS, the US government, and the Clinton Foundation. Former US president Bill Clinton called the program "a model for any country that wants to increase the efficiency of foreign aid and improve the health of its people." Some of global health's heavyweights were finally in the ring.

In many ways the Rwandan model was the kind of comprehensive training campaign Dilan had long hoped Madaktari Africa would pull off. Except for the Henry Jackson Foundation grant, Madaktari hadn't had a big push. It remained a loose network of mostly volunteer doctors and nurses. Paid a dollar, D Word did his best to move the program forward. Dilan was up to his lobes in aneurysm and stroke patients. And his life at home also had gathered force, though in an entirely different way.

Sixteen months after giving birth to Else, Carin had a son, Dauwe. Soon, a third was on the way, a girl they would name Calla. Then, as the months passed, he grew frustrated with what he thought was the slow pace of MUSC's neurosurgery department, a rerun of Oregon. Dilan knew that some at MUSC were leery about the time he spent on his global health work, even as it brought the department national attention. And he could be difficult. At home, he was tender and goofy. But at work he was sometimes short with people he thought weren't on his side or who asked questions he thought they could answer themselves. He'd burned through several assistants.

As he mulled over his future, Centra Health, a nonprofit hospital system in Lynchburg, Virginia, offered him a chance to create a neuroscience institute. He thought about how John Jane at the University of Virginia had trained him to be a department chairman. He imagined what it might be like to have fewer layers of management over his head.

In late 2011 the growing Ellegala clan moved from South Carolina to a leafy old neighborhood in Lynchburg. His parents moved into a house behind theirs. His father, Somisara, was in his nineties now, working on a book about Buddhism, and using a broom handle to walk around. Dilan's mother, Chitra, cooked Sri Lankan curries with coconut rice and jackfruit. Carin planted a small *shamba* farm with sunflowers that grew twelve feet high. They built a chicken coop and raised ducks. It was their own little *boma*.

As he had at MUSC, Dilan persuaded colleagues at Centra to join him in his overseas work. In 2013 Centra created two global health fellowships to send residents to teach neurosurgery in Dar es Salaam and Haydom for six months. Other Centra doctors flew to Dar es Salaam to train staff in the new heart catheter lab. Several MUSC employees moved to Lynchburg, as did a neurosurgeon from the Barrow. Dilan could be difficult, but he was a pied piper.

As the years passed, Madaktari Africa coordinated teaching programs that taught dozens of doctors in Tanzania when the country needed thousands. Meantime, the need for more surgeons across the world had only grown. Building on Haile Debas's earlier findings, other researchers calculated that 17 million people died every year from conditions that could have been treated with surgery. That was many times more than the 1.4 million lives lost to AIDS and 1.2

million lives lost to malaria. And with more cars and trucks on the roads, developing countries such as Tanzania would only see more trauma cases in the coming years.

The need was there, and Madaktari Africa was in the thick of this issue, but Dilan and D Word occasionally found themselves sidetracked by activities that had little to do with training, such as helping MUSC donate secondhand library books to a medical school in Tanzania, exactly the kind of thing they wanted to move away from. They spent precious time showing potential donors around Haydom, including one wealthy woman who merely donated the suitcase she bought for the trip. Doing these kinds of things made them sometimes wonder if their mission had gotten fuzzy.

On one visit in early 2013, Dilan and D Word were in the lobby of the Arusha Hotel, in Dar es Salaam, talking about Madaktari's future. Emanuel Nuwas joined them just after twilight. Storm clouds gathered around Mount Meru. Nuwas had driven from Moshi where he was doing his advanced surgical training. His wife had just given birth to a daughter, he said, his eyes narrowing in a weary smile. Someday when she was to be married, he would give away a single calf and twenty liters of honey. The honey would be brewed into an alcoholic beverage for everyone to share. As he talked, his eyes grew heavier with fatigue. He had operated through the night until 5 a.m. Dilan gave him a knowing smile. Pressure makes the best surgeons. Good for him. Good for Nuwas's future patients.

But Nuwas had mixed feelings about having left Haydom. He'd passed the scalpel to Hayte Samo, but then Hayte also decided to seek surgical training. Hayte had tried to find someone else in Haydom to replace him; he wanted to teach the surgical techniques he'd learned from Nuwas and Dilan. But none of the new doctors and interns had the right mix of intelligence and focus. Surgery wasn't something you could force on someone, and Hayte had left Haydom with a heavy heart. The chain had been broken. Once again, patients with neurological problems would depend on the odd chance that a foreign surgeon was visiting. People would die because they had failed to teach another doctor.

As Nuwas spoke, he put his hands together like a professor, forefinger to forefinger, thumb to thumb. Then his voice rose, just a few decibels, but enough to draw Dilan's eyes toward his. The government and the medical community should find a way to certify the hands-on surgical experience they received in Haydom. Clinicians and young doctors should be rewarded for their initiative. A program that certified doctors based on experience rather than years in medical school or residency would speed more surgeons into the field. Lives would be saved.

Exactly, Dilan thought.

Later, after Nuwas left, Dilan and D Word took seats around a table on the hotel's patio. The power went out, as it did many nights. Above, stars poked through the haze. Thinking about Nuwas, Dilan's mind lit up like heat lightning.

Nuwas had cut to the marrow: the William Halsted residency model of building surgeons wasn't the only option. Halsted and his colleagues developed the rigorous program to weed out incompetent and uneducated practitioners. The residency model had been a brilliant innovation in the late 1800s, but the world needed lots of doctors now. It takes about fourteen years to mint a surgeon in the United States. Surely there were other options. Nuwas was talking about teaching essential surgeries and certifying their qualifications along the way.

"He's thinking about curriculum and certification," Dilan said. "He's gone two steps beyond the things I've thought about. He has the answers, not us. That's success. That's special. That's what we want to achieve with everyone." Nuwas wasn't just a surgeon, he was a leader.

"Great, so we're successful in Haydom, and now we can go away," D Word joked, then got serious. "I like what you say about ownership."

"Ownership and leadership," Dilan added.

"It dies without both," D Word said.

"Exactly. To take it to the next level, we need to find these key individuals."

"You know," Dilan continued, "you can look online now and find a thousand other NGOs saying 'sustainable' and 'teach a man to fish.'"

"And now you even hear people talking about an exit strategy," D piped in.

"We need to be clear about what we do," Dilan said, growing excited. "This is an epiphany for me. Teach a man to fish is not enough. Our job is to cultivate leaders to teach. That would be huge."

Moments later, the power came back on.

This was the direction he wanted to take the program in the coming years: identify and cultivate medical leaders to train others. Other activities should take a back seat. He rubbed his eyes and said nothing for what seemed like three minutes but was thirty seconds.

"I'll tell you one thing," he said finally. "Madaktari is a failure if Nuwas, Mayegga, and Hayte don't return to Haydom and create their own sustainable training program."

He didn't know at the time, but Haydom Lutheran Hospital was about to confront a sustainability crisis of its own.

CHAPTER 49

In early 2013 the rainy season came on time, turning gullies around Mount Haydom into serpentine sluices. Brown water poured onto the plateau, and farmers tended patches of sunflowers and maize. In Haydom town, teenage boys and girls waited by the water tank to fill their yellow jugs. Nearby, young men turned broken black bicycles upside down for repairs. Sounds of hammers and wrenches blended with radios playing Afro-beat. Music came from small kiosks where shopkeepers sold mangos and airtime for mobile phones. Rainy season was a time to plant, gather, and fix.

After his day at the hospital, Baba Naman took a seat on the patio of his wife's restaurant and listened to Haydom's twilight chorus: the crickets, the voices of people walking home, the day's exhalation. Mama Naman appeared in the door, set a plate of vegetables in front of him, and then took it away at the last second, a little joke. He looked at her with a twinkle in his eye as she set it down again and rested her hand on his shoulder. Night fell, stars poured out, and the sounds of the crickets swelled and receded like waves. The waves, row on row, merged with the hoof thumps of cattle and goats being moved into *bomas*, the sharp barks of dogs, and an occasional hyena howl. Then in the distance, people began yelling, "*Ohayoda! Ohayoda!*" And soon everyone knew that a five-year-old girl was lost.

The girl would be returned to her *boma* in a few hours, found by the night cries and a neighbor. As Baba Naman sat there, he wondered about Emmanuel Mayegga. Would he return to Haydom? Mayegga was nearing the end of medical school in Dar es Salaam. He missed Mayegga's company on the patio. Even when Mayegga had one beer too many and got all worked up. Baba Naman would listen and let the storm pass, and then they would talk about things that mattered. He was confident that Mayegga would keep his promise to the hospital, but living so far away and for so long can rewire a person. He would wait for this man, whom he had come to love as a son.

Then, as the months passed and the rainy season ended, the acacias dropped their leaves to conserve water. The air lost its humidity, and now everything was sharp and bright and hot. The winds picked up, spawning the brown twisters on the plateau. The red soil dried, and the dust on the road to Haydom town felt like ground chalk. The earth underneath the dust hardened, so much that ants climbed into the whistling thorn acacias and built bulbous nests. The ants drilled tiny holes in these nests, and when the wind blew, the bulbs whistled like flutes. The sun grew hotter, and the ground cracked under its glare. More patients were admitted for malnutrition, tuberculosis, pneumonia, parasites, and other diseases that preyed on weakness. Dry season was a time of reckoning, a time to give up or move forward. Winds flung the chalky dust into the air. The hospital's reckoning had come.

Would Haydom Lutheran Hospital close?

For so long, such a thought wouldn't have crossed anyone's mind. The hospital's first buildings had gone up with all the optimism and possibility that accompany any new birth. During the hospital's adolescence, everything was about growth, expansion— the future. But now, in late 2013 and nearing the hospital's sixtieth anniversary, the possibility of its demise didn't seem so far-fetched. True, it was one of the largest rural hospitals in Tanzania, the health care hub for a region of nearly two million people—indispensable. But it was still a missionary hospital funded largely by people five thousand miles away.

Questions about the hospital's future had simmered for years but began to boil after 2010. That year Oystein Olsen, the third Dr. Olsen, returned to Norway with his family, including his mother, Mama Kari. For the first time in generations, an Olsen didn't live full time on the grounds.

Another Norwegian replaced Oystein, a gentle, silver-haired missionary in his late sixties named Olav Espegren. A psychiatrist by training, Espegren arrived in late 2010 with his equally silver-haired wife, Turid. Espegren had worked in Haydom for four years in the early 1970s and then gone on to do missionary work in Hong Kong. In Haydom once again, Espegren found the hospital in disarray. Records were missing. There had been thefts of gas from the garage and allegations of stolen construction materials. At least $42,000 had been embezzled from an American HIV/AIDS treatment fund. Four people in the finance department were fired. Shipping containers of donated equipment were still strewn across the compound. The hospital still had no inventory of their contents. Curious, Turid began searching through them. In one she found a washing machine from Europe with a tag that roughly translated to "Send to Haydom, Beyond Repair." Increasingly that seemed to be the case for the hospital itself.

Then in 2013, while in Dar es Salaam, Olav Espegren fell down a flight of stairs. He and Anderson Sakweli had traveled to the city to meet with President Kikwete and government health officials about the hospital's future. At the time, the hospital was nearing the end of its five-year grant from Norway, with no promise yet of renewal.

Dilan and D Word were also in Tanzania at the time and had planned to join Espegren and Sakweli at the State House for fish and *ugali* with the president. After hearing about Espegren's fall, they rushed to a small private hospital on Barack Obama Drive. They found Espegren in the ICU, barely conscious from a severe head injury. Dilan examined Espegren and looked at an X-ray.

"He should be OK, but it will take some time to heal," Dilan said.

Concerned about the level of care in Tanzania, Espegren's family whisked him back to Norway to recuperate.

Without a medical director, Haydom Lutheran Hospital continued to drift. Salary payments were delayed; visa money from foreign doctors went missing; the operating theaters closed one Friday because they ran out of sutures. Mayegga, Nuwas, and Hayte were still away but tried to keep up with the turn of events. "When the adults are away, the cattle leave the *boma*," Nuwas said one afternoon, citing a local proverb.

Communication between the hospital and Norwegian leaders all but ceased. In this vacuum, factions in Norway questioned why the government should keep pumping money into such a faraway hospital. No one could say whether the grant money, like the rainy season, would return. A handful of Norwegian volunteers and foreign doctors grew so concerned that they launched a crowdfunding campaign to make a documentary, *Life Without Care: Losing Haydom Hospital.*

The months passed, and the end of the grant money grew near. High clouds appeared in the sky and let a few drops go, but the rain didn't come. In Mama Naman's restaurant, Baba Naman and his friends gathered around the television at night. After the news, he sat with friends and talked of the past—how the area around Haydom once had zebras, giraffes, and other wild game, even into the 1980s, but now you could find such animals only in the Yaida Chini Valley where the Hadza people lived. It had been nearly sixty years since the leopard attacked the hospital's construction workers, forcing the first Dr. Olsen to break out the sutures. The hospital's sixtieth anniversary would be celebrated in January 2015. If the hospital survived, there would be a big party, for sure.

CHAPTER 50

Hayte Samo had promised he would return to Haydom after his surgical training in Dar es Salaam. But sometimes he thought it made more sense, in purely financial terms, to stay in the city. When he completed his training, he could set up a private surgical practice. His skills would be in great demand. He would earn much more money, enough to help more friends and family. And now that he was a doctor, they expected this: if you had food or money, you shared it. This had long been the Datoga way. You never knew when you might need something as well. But salaries in Haydom and other rural hospitals in Tanzania were thin; he would be hard-pressed to meet people's expectations, unless, perhaps, he stayed in Dar es Salaam.

Yet, in early October 2013 he found himself back on the plateau, although not because of his promise to Haydom Lutheran Hospital. He returned to bury his father.

Gastric cancer had finally cut him down. Such a tough old tree. His *baba* was maybe ninety years old, maybe a hundred. No one knew. What the Datoga people knew for sure was his place in history, particularly as a peacemaker. After his death the community had agreed to hold a *bung'eda*, a funeral reserved for only the most respected Datoga men.

The *bung'eda* had begun in March, soon after his father's death. Hayte and his people smeared his father's body in butter. They folded his arms and legs into a seated position, knees to chest, and tied them in place with a leather strap. They draped a fresh cattle hide around his father's shoulders and lowered him into a grave, making sure his body faced east so he would forever watch the rising sun.

Hayte and his father had drifted apart during his school days, but the pull of time and blood had brought them together again. Hayte's stature had grown within the Datoga community because he was a doctor, which enhanced the reputation of the entire family. And Hayte had also taken care to respect Datoga traditions. When he visited his father's *boma*, he removed his Western clothes and wore a *shuka* blanket. He grabbed a staff and helped herd the goats. He spoke Datoga, not Swahili. During Hayte's visits, his *baba* sometimes grew sad.

"I am ashamed," he told Hayte one day. "I don't have a proper bed for you to sleep on."

"I am still the same Hayte, your son," Hayte replied. He didn't need a mattress; a cattle hide was perfectly fine. A few years before he died, his father told him with a distant gaze, "I wish I could be young again, so all of my children could have gone to school like you."

In the months after his father's death, people from across the plateau brought sticks and mud to the grave. Over time it grew into a large conical tomb, grayish brown like the soil around it. A rope was placed around the tomb to symbolize a belt. Midway was a hole that resembled a navel. People poured milk and honey into the hole to feed the *baba's* spirit. A patch of sod was placed on the top, symbolizing hair. By October the tomb was twice as tall as Hayte.

On October 12, the final day of the *bung'eda*, more than one thousand people from across the region gathered around the tomb. Women wore tasseled goatskin skirts and covered their arms with brass bracelets. Men drank *gesoda*, a hearty brew made from juices extracted from roots of aloe vera and blended with honey. The dry-season sun had baked moisture from the tomb's outer layer, leaving it cracked like an old man's skin. A group of men led a cow to the tomb. The men placed their hands around the animal's mouth to suffocate it, and the cow went down quietly, a sign that the *baba* in the tomb was a good man.

People screamed louder, as if in ecstasy and pain. The chorus swelled and then suddenly grew silent as a Datoga elder led Hayte through the crowd. Around his shoulders, Hayte wore a piece of cattle hide that had been softened with butter. His chest was bare. He removed the hide when he reached the tomb and used several logs to climb to the top.

He gazed at the crowd, which covered every inch around the tomb and spilled down a dirt road. With a microphone in one hand, he spoke about the importance of his people's traditions. He said a prayer in Datoga: "May God bless this man and us, so that we will live as long as he had, and live our lives as he had, helping people, and become people of good repute."

He planted a sapling on the cap of the tomb. Over time the tree would sprout and grow, even as the tomb below shrank. He stood high above the body of his father.

He had made his decision.

He would return to Haydom Lutheran Hospital when he finished his surgical training.

He would do it for his father's people, who spread out like a large circular *shuka* round the tomb. As he looked at them he felt an even deeper love for his father. For the first time he truly experienced the burdens his father had carried, because suddenly they were his.

A few days after the *bung'eda*, a Nyaturu boy named Paulo was hunting with friends near Singida. Because it was the end of dry season, the grass was yellow-white, the trees were bare, and a strong wind blew. They threw large sticks into the air, including one that flew high and down into Paulo's forehead.

The stick struck with such force that it went through his skull and lodged in his brain. Somehow his family found a way to get him to Iambic Hospital, a small missionary hospital near Singida. But the clinician there could do nothing for him but load him on a truck to Haydom with a note: "Brain protruded out of the skull bone." He spent the evening in a corner of Haydom Lutheran Hospital's ICU, unconscious, his body jerking from the trauma.

The next morning, a German medical student named Jonas Scheck stood at his bed, wondering what would happen to the boy.

Clearly, Paulo needed surgery. With an open wound like that, his brain would certainly become infected. But as far as Scheck knew, the hospital didn't have a neurosurgeon.

Then a man walked into the ICU. He wore a long white doctor's coat. He had a serious look on his face, a thin mustache, and a high hairline that made his forehead stand out.

His nametag said "Dr. Mayegga."

It was Emmanuel Mayegga's second day back at the hospital after finishing medical school. He had that slightly nervous and joyful feeling of returning to a familiar place after a long time—unsure of how it had changed and how he had changed as well.

He'd spent so many years in Dar es Salaam in that small corner in the stairwell studying his medical texts. He had taken so many exams, made so many long trips from Dar es Salaam to Haydom to see his wife, Samwayma, and children, Godwin, Godlisten, and Glory. His grades hadn't been good at the beginning, but he was near the top of his class by the end.

He'd heard about the Nyaturu boy during morning report. He was slightly irritated with the intern who recited the case. The intern hadn't been clear. Mayegga had heard only "head injury" and "occipital area." The intern should have been more specific. Was it a closed head injury? Was it open? Was it severe, mild, or moderate? He would have to teach him.

In the ICU, he leaned over Paulo. The boy couldn't talk but responded to Mayegga's palpations. Good sign. "Occipital area" meant the injury was in the back of the boy's head. He turned the boy's head for a look. *Nothing there. Where is this thing? Had the intern mixed up his anatomy?* He peeled off the bandage on the boy's forehead. There it was: the hole where the stick had entered, the dura bloody and red, and a few bits of brain tissue, pinkish-white, spilling out.

"We have to close this wound," he said to Jonas Scheck as much as to himself. *Time is brain.*

"How long will the procedure take?" Scheck asked.

"It can be just five minutes," Mayegga said. "But if it's complicated, it can be two hours." If he cared to observe, he'd show him how it was done.

When Mayegga entered the theater, everyone welcomed him with hugs and smiles, and Jonas Scheck wondered whether these warm greetings were typical before surgeries in Tanzania. Mayegga explained, "It is my first time back in the theater in many years."

Mayegga put a green cotton cap on his head and scrubbed his hands. He walked into Theater One and said a prayer. Would he remember what to do?

He picked up a No. 10 scalpel and made a C-shaped cut, a large arc to create a flap. The cut was uneven. *I'm out of practice—all that book learning.* Rust on the old neural pathways.

Another incision. Better.

Now, drill a hole with the Hudson Brace. Good.

Then something inside his mind broke free, and once again the blade felt familiar, and he could lose himself in the artistry of moving through human tissue. And then there it was, the brain, exposed and pulsating, the boy's future. He used a needlelike instrument to remove a skull fragment. He spotted an artery. No clots, good news. No cerebral spinal fluid leaking, more good news. He cleaned the dirt out of the boy's brain and closed with 2.0 Vicryl sutures, three stitches. Wound dressed, bandage applied. Done in just over an hour. A brain surgeon once again.

Four days after the hospital discharged the Nyaturu boy, Mayegga was at home nailing a piece of wood when he smashed his thumb. The finger throbbed; he'd lose the nail for sure, but at least his finger wasn't broken. He canceled a hernia and some other minor procedures, but one patient needed surgery immediately: an older woman with a brain abscess. He would do it one-handed.

Outside, the sky was gray as he walked toward the hospital's administration building. Clouds had come and gone again that morning, leaving a few raindrops. The rainy season was near. By the administration building, he spotted an older man in a gray suit and a beanie hat with OBAMA stitched on the front. His name was Zacharia Munya. Munya and his family were the only people who lived by Mount Haydom when the Norwegians arrived so long ago. Munya's mother had just died, and he was making burial arrangements now. Holding his injured thumb, Mayegga nodded toward Munya and then spotted an old friend.

Emanuel Nuwas turned the corner.

Nuwas was back for a holiday break. His face was a little plumper than when he'd started his surgical residency, but his eyes still had the same focus and mirth. He wore a dark blue shirt with a shiny finish. He greeted Mayegga with a warm handshake, and Mayegga showed off his injured thumb. At least it was on his left hand, he said. "I've canceled all my elective surgeries, but I will try to help this woman."

"I would be happy to assist," Nuwas said, a Tanzanian way of saying, "No worries, I'll do the surgery instead."

Side by side, they went to Radiology to make a plan. Nuwas held a mobile phone in his left hand; Mayegga's coat billowed like a white cape. They found the CT room empty but with the lights on. Nuwas took a seat at the computer and clicked the mouse. The computer wasn't working, so he tried the backup. No problem. The CT scans appeared. Mayegga leaned over his shoulder.

"I'll make one incision here," Nuwas said. "I'll drill the holes here and here, one, two." Two jabs with his fingers. Done. Mayegga could go and do his rounds. He had backup.

In Theater One, masked and gowned, Nuwas prepared the Hudson Brace. A new Tanzanian doctor scrubbed in. "That's good," Nuwas told him. "I always like to teach, to leave something behind in my absence."

The woman was on her back. Her arms were spread wide on two wooden planks as if she were about to be crucified. Nuwas took the drill and cranked the handle.

"You have to be very careful," he told the young doctor. A few seconds later, the bit broke and lodged in the woman's skull; blood formed around the burr hole. Nuwas's fingers moved quickly to bring it under control.

"Sometimes it's good for people to see mistakes," he said. He drilled another hole, flushed the woman's brain with saline. "You can see the clots drain now."

In the hallway afterward, the doctor asked Nuwas if he would help him with a case in Lena Ward.

"Of course," Nuwas said.

They walked under the jacaranda trees and into the empty play-room of the Lena Ward. Through the double doors and in a room on the left they found a *mama* holding her baby girl tight. The girl had hydrocephalus. Nuwas held her up and examined her back. She also had spina bifida. The baby's vomiting had gotten worse; she needed a VP shunt.

"Would you do the procedure, Dr. Nuwas? Please let's not have this patient bear the cost of going to Arusha. Please let us save this woman's baby."

"Yes, of course," Nuwas said. It was his vacation, but what is that compared to the suffering of a *mama* and her baby? "Let's be sure we have the shunt," he said. The Tanzanian doctor nodded and said, "Dr. Nuwas and Dr. Mayegga are the keys to this hospital's future."

Nuwas left the Lena Ward to have a bite in the staff canteen. On his way, the family member of a patient greeted him and asked a few questions about a loved one. The consultation over, Nuwas had taken only a few steps before a clinical officer approached to ask about a case. Nuwas answered with patience and good humor, went to the canteen, gobbled down *ugali* and chicken, then plunged into the theater again, like those twisters he'd run into so long ago. No foreign doctors in sight.

CHAPTER 51

The rainy season finally came, and with it news that Haydom Lutheran Hospital would keep its doors open. A wealthy Norwegian had left money for the hospital in his estate, and that money bought the hospital time. Then, as the Norwegian block grant was about to run out, the Norwegian government agreed to give the hospital another push—a four-year block grant instead of the five-year grant it had committed to in the past.

Political support for the hospital remained strong in southern Norway, where the Olsens and other missionary families still made their homes. But questions circled like buzzards: As the old missionary families died, would that support continue? And why would the Norwegian government continue to spend so much money on a hospital in another hemisphere?

In the short term, the hospital would survive to celebrate its sixtieth jubilee. It would be one of the biggest celebrations since the wedding on the airstrip. Hundreds of people gathered under the jacaranda trees between the chapel and the outpatient clinic. Norway's ambassador to Tanzania listened to the velvet sounds of the hospital choir. The hospital rented rows of plastic chairs from a catering company that Mama Naman had started with the other village *mamas*. The staff performed a skit in the Old Ward. They reenacted the hospital's birth, including a scene where the leopard mauled four construction workers and a Norwegian shot the leopard dead. Emanuel Nuwas, done with his surgical training, starred as the first Dr. Olsen.

Olav and Turid Espegren were in Haydom for the jubilee and to say good-bye. His head injury had been severe, and his Norwegian doctors feared that Haydom's mile-high altitude might affect the chemical balance in his brain. Two days after the jubilee, he and Turid left Haydom for their home in Norway.

This time a Tanzanian doctor would take over: Emanuel Nuwas.

With Nuwas in the director's office, a wave of relief washed through the compound, with all the optimism and uncertainty that comes with a fresh start. Staff spoke with pride about having a Tanzanian director, but some also longed for the days of the second Dr. Olsen. Now that the Olsen days had passed, that time had a certainty about it that the future could never match.

Nuwas plunged into his new role with his usual confidence, sensitivity, and feelings of responsibility. His mind spun with ideas: teaching would be the key to the hospital's future; someday it could be the site of a university hospital; the country desperately needed to keep doctors in rural areas, so why not use Haydom Lutheran Hospital as a model? With its buildings for all the foreign doctors, it already had the feel of a campus. *Anything is possible*, he thought. Proof? All he had to do was look around at the people he was working with now.

Emmanuel Mayegga was back in the theaters doing one procedure after another. And Hayte Samo had just returned from his surgical residency in Dar es Salaam. And a half dozen other Tanzanian doctors who had sought residency-level training were also back in Haydom or on their way. A year before, the hospital had no Tanzanian specialists. Now it would have six, including a Tanzanian pediatrician in the Lena Ward. Now during morning meetings the foreign students sat in the rear, and Mayegga and Hayte sat in the front near the light board. When a Dutch doctor asked about brain scans, she directed the questions to them: "What do the neurosurgeons think?"

CHAPTER 52

In Lynchburg one November morning, Carin moved from kitchen counter to child. Calla sat in her high chair, holding her head in a royal way, eyeing Else and Dauwe, who giggled and fidgeted as they waited for breakfast. Dauwe shouted "No!" because it had mysterious powers to command attention. Suddenly they turned to look at their father, who walked in wearing his long black overcoat. The children looked up with grins as he kissed their mother, and then them, and said he would see them all that night.

Dilan opened the back door and inhaled. The cool late autumn air had a hint of burned leaves. The sky was a layer of white against pale blue. He was off to the hospital to operate on a nurse who had a giant aneurysm between her frontal and left temporal lobes. To fix it, he and his team would perform a standstill, the same operation he did with Arthur Day at Harvard eight years before. As far as he knew, it was the first standstill ever attempted in Virginia. He hoped that this time the patient would survive.

Her name was Shannon Frazier. She'd been in a bad car wreck some months before, and her doctors discovered the aneurysm while treating her other injuries. Since she was a nurse, she knew that an aneurysm this size was a death sentence. The only question was when it would rupture. Her headaches grew worse. She felt as if someone were driving ice picks into her ears. She sobbed when it got too bad. "Someone make it stop." She heard that a doctor named Ellegala in Lynchburg, Virginia, not far from her home, might be able to help.

When Dilan saw the aneurysm's size and location, he knew Shannon's only hope was a standstill.

She'd asked, "What are my chances of surviving this operation?"

He looked her straight in the eye.

"Fifty-fifty."

"Have you ever done a standstill before?" she asked.

"Yes."

"How were those outcomes?"

"Not good." He kept it at that.

She'd asked him what she should do, and he knew she wanted him to decide for her. Most patients did.

Instead, he told her the aneurysm could rupture tomorrow or in five years. She would have headaches in the meantime. "You can live with headaches." But a standstill operation could be fatal. She would have to make the decision, but before she did, she should take six weeks and think about it.

He could tell she was surprised. A surgeon who doesn't want to operate? But he wanted her to own the decision. If she survived, she would forever know she had the courage to save herself.

When the six weeks were up, she'd said, "I can't live with a time bomb in my head anymore. And I don't want my family to suddenly find me dead one day."

She needed help, and he was her last hope.

He climbed into his old white pickup. The transmission wasn't working properly, and he had to drive in second gear to a nearby Starbucks. Surgery has unwritten rules, and one of the first is to maintain your routine the day of a big operation. Since medical school, he had trained his muscles and nervous system to work on one large cup of coffee in the morning. Less, and you get a withdrawal headache. More, and your hands might shake.

He drove through Lynchburg's rolling hills toward the hospital. The drive gave him time to settle his mind—get those butterflies to fly in formation, think about what had gone wrong before and what had gone right.

. . .

That standstill eight years before at Harvard was a failure but also a gift. It cemented his plan to go to Africa for six months, no matter what it cost his career. That, in turn, had led to his discovery of a neglected global health problem, the shortage of surgeons, and his decision to teach Mayegga, who taught Nuwas, who taught Hayte. Before, brain surgery patients in Haydom had no hope. Now, these three doctors were doing more than one hundred brain surgeries a year—and getting better. He and Joyce Nicholas, a researcher who moved from Charleston to Lynchburg because of Dilan's work, had studied their performances. Their complication rates were going down even as the complexity of the procedures went up. The results eventually were published in the *Journal of Neurosurgery*, just as Dilan had predicted to Nuwas in 2010. It was proof that his model worked.

President Jakaya Kikwete remained a staunch supporter of Madaktari Africa and delighted in talking about Dilan's work with Mayegga. "Here is a man who is a clinician, an assistant medical officer, and he becomes a neurosurgeon. How about that?" Kikwete said one evening after a meeting at the United Nations in New York. "It's something very innovative. But he's there. He's saving lives." Tanzania itself had made efforts to increase the number of doctors. In 2006, the year Dilan first arrived in Haydom, its medical schools were graduating 250 doctors a year. Now they were producing more than 1,500. It was still not enough. Canada, with fewer people than Tanzania, graduated about 2,500 doctors a year. But ripples can form waves once they cross and join with each other.

He and Carin would see those waves form in Haydom three weeks after the sixtieth jubilee. They flew to Tanzania with Else, Dauwe, and Calla and set up house in a cottage with a view of Mount Hanang. In Lena Ward, Nurse Angela stretched out her arms and screamed with joy when she saw Carin. Carin smiled so much as she did rounds that her face ached by the end of the day.

Carin worked in Lena Ward during the mornings, doing what she could but keeping it in balance. When she finished, she returned to the cottage full of energy and light. Meantime, Dilan played with the children or tinkered with his old green Land Rover, which had been passed from one doctor to another in his absence. Some nights he had long talks with Emanuel Nuwas about his new role as medical director. Nuwas confessed that he was struggling to balance his desire to do surgery and fulfill his administrative duties. As the weeks passed, though, Dilan saw something take root inside Nuwas. Nuwas spoke about how he wanted to emulate the second Dr. Olsen, who had made a point of talking to all the staff, from the guards to the cleaners. And Nuwas would continue to operate, just as the old Norwegian had done in his day. He would do his best to be the next Dr. Olsen.

Dilan had equally long talks with Hayte Samo, who also was thinking hard about the future. Many had urged him to get into politics. "I don't want to lie, so how can I be a politician?" he said. But Dilan saw a change in Hayte during his visit, new neural connections that made Hayte decide, yes, he could do even more for his people if he ran for a seat in Parliament.

And Emmanuel Mayegga was leading in his own way, settling into his role as a busy doctor and thinking about where in Haydom to build a new house. On the patio with Baba Naman, he and Dilan talked about making Haydom Lutheran Hospital an international neurosurgery training site. Mayegga's horizon was still moving outward, as the moon did when Dilan and Carin walked back to the hospital from Mama Naman's restaurant. "They are all taking true leadership paths," Dilan had said. And one morning in the theaters he had seen no better example.

Mayegga was in Theater One, operating on an elderly man with a tumor in his frontal lobe.

In Theater Two, Hayte operated on a man with cysticercosis, a parasite from improperly cooked pork; the parasite had worked its way into the man's brain and created cysts that looked like clusters of grapes.

"Two brain surgeries at the same time!" Dilan said out loud. In a country that a few years before had only three brain surgeons, total. Even more important: that morning Mayegga and Hayte taught another young Tanzanian doctor with great potential. And two college students—the twin sons of the Tanzanian prime minister—observed.

One of the sons later said with pride how he wanted to be a neuro-surgeon one day.

Afterward, Dilan had said, "This is the completion of a cycle for me. They're all doing neurosurgery. They're all leaders, but they're leading in different ways. They're showing what happens when people change the way they think about themselves. They're showing what happens when you break from a normal path, what happens inside an individual, and how that can affect so many others."

During walks to the airstrip in twilight's amber hues, or on the porch in the mornings as the sun rose to the left of Hanang, Dilan and Carin talked about spending more time in nature, about buying a van in the States, camping together in parks, a merry little band. Dilan would work on groundbreaking neurosurgery ventures, but he'd probably never be the chairman of a neurosurgery department, which was fine. Belonging and family were more lasting than achievement. They both had chosen love over individual dreams and career advancement, and even their global health work, but the result was the way they held each other in their eyes, the way they knew their children, and how their children knew them. There was a heavy downpour one afternoon, though not quite as rough as the one on their wedding, and Else grinned and ran out the door. She told her father she was going to take an outside shower, because that's what he had done when he was a child in Sri Lanka. He watched her dance in the rain and thought, *I have a life.*

At Starbucks, Dilan bought his coffee and felt the liquid warm his hands. He took a curvy two-lane road to Centra, which sat in a dip just above Blackwater Creek. He pulled into Centra's parking lot just after 7 a.m. and took a side door inside. Through a quiet lobby, he took a stairway to a long hallway of paneled wood, where he heard someone cry out. *I think that's my patient.*

He found Shannon Frazier on a gurney, surrounded by nurses. She was having a panic attack—understandable given what was about to happen. He watched the nurses calm her. Satisfied that they had things under control, he changed into his scrubs. It seemed oddly quiet as he collapsed into a comfortable leather chair. *Oh, shit, it's Friday.* On Fridays, they started surgeries an hour later than normal. He could have slept in a bit, a crushing blow. "No one told me," he said to a nurse.

"We did that so you would show up on time," she replied.

Another nurse popped her head through the door. "The patient wants to talk to you."

He walked through the OR control room into pre-op. He opened a movable curtain. Shannon was now properly sedated.

"Can you give me an extra pill?" she joked. "And how about throwing in a little plastic surgery while I'm under?" Dilan let her talk, and then her eyes grew moist.

"Do you have a plan?" she asked.

"Yes, I have a plan."

He scrubbed in, taking twice as long as usual. No time for chit-chat with a doctor next to him. Time to get in the game. Those perforator vessels would be difficult to see. Cut one, and she has a stroke or is paralyzed or dies. Nearby, a scrub nurse said to another, "I'm so excited. This is history."

The OR felt like a meat locker when he stepped inside—temperature at sixty-six degrees and going down. He'd worn long underwear but was still cold, so he wrapped a warming blanket around his torso.

"Must be why he likes Tanzania so much," a technician said.

Fourteen people moved around the patient like planes around an airport. They readied instrument trays, checked equipment, manned monitors. Dilan helped place Shannon's head in a Mayfield clamp, tightening screws into her skull. Shannon all but disappeared under blue surgical drapes.

It's on. He took a purple marker and drew a line on the shaved part of her scalp. With a No. 10 scalpel, he made the first cut. He used an electric saw to cut open her skull. He exchanged it for a scalpel. He sliced through the dura, exposing her brain. He brought the microscope to his eyes; time to peel apart the lobes. Forceps and suckers, spread, suck, spread. A video monitor showed his progress. Deeper into her brain, spread, suck, spread.

Then, there it was, the aneurysm, pink with white striations from the plaque.

"Hey, guys," he said in a pilot's calm voice. "If the aneurysm tears now, we're going to have catastrophic bleeding."

The heart and lung team went about their business; the nurses said nothing.

"Hey, did you guys hear me?" Quick muffled nods of assent. *OK, they're on it.*

Her pulse was sixty. With his forceps, he positioned the aneurysm. His foot tapped.

"You guys are great. Everything you see here is an aneurysm," he said, teaching. "You still can't see around it. This is either the back side of the aneurysm or the branch vessel, which I can't see unless we decompress it. Call Dr. Frantz." The heart surgeon. Frantz and his team made a one-inch incision in the groin area and punctures in the neck. A directional light on the blue surgical drapes cast the room in an eerie tint. Her body temperature plunged to fifty-seven degrees. Her heartbeat slowed because of the cold. Then her heart fibrillated and stopped. The squiggles on the brain wave monitor went flat.

Standstill.

The blood pressure: "Let's lower it to thirty and see what we can see." At Harvard, they'd gone to zero. Not this time. He would keep the blood pressure up. Forgive, now remember.

He looked through the microscope. Everything had opened up. He could see around the aneurysm. He knew what to avoid and where to put the clip.

"I gotta tell you, the view here is spectacular!"

In this moment of stillness, the path was clear. He could save her now, and he would.

In a world of trauma and disease, destinies are often shaped by access to healers. And without this access, ripples of suffering can become waves. Consider what happened in late 2014 in the West African country of Guinea. A two-year-old boy developed a fever. Then his family members fell ill, and soon so did people in his village.

No one thought about Ebola as villagers buried their dead. The most recent outbreak had been in Uganda. But within several months the virus had spread beyond Guinea to Sierra Leone and Liberia. Like a weak immune system, the health-care systems in these countries would be no match.

Before the outbreak, Liberia had just two hundred doctors to care for its population of four million. When it came to doctor-patient ratios, Liberia was way below the first rung. But fifteen other sub-Saharan African countries, including Tanzania, were only a tad higher. In Liberia's case, most of its two hundred physicians were expats. Roughly fifty physicians were from Liberia, fewer than you might find in a single North American teaching hospital. The country had just three Liberian surgeons.

As the Ebola cases multiplied, humanitarian groups faced gut-wrenching decisions: Should they keep their doctors there or send them home? "We need you guys here," the Liberian nurses and doctors told one group. A few expat doctors stayed, and a few contracted the disease. The first three Americans to contract Ebola were Christian medical mission workers, one of whom died. But nearly 95 percent of the foreign health-care workers packed their bags. Hospitals and clinics closed; the disease spread to Nigeria,

Mali, Senegal, and then the United States and Spain. West Africa's problem became the world's problem.

Headlines were written about a horrible epidemic, but the real story was about a much deeper failure. As Dilan and a growing number of health leaders might have predicted, decades of humanitarian work, often with the best of intentions, had failed to create health-care systems that could stand on their own. Worse, like a hidden virus, Western countries had contributed to this failure by siphoning doctors from poor countries to shore up their own health-care workforces.

The Ebola crisis also came amid a growing consensus in international health circles: Haile Debas, Atul Gawande, Paul Farmer, and other leaders in this arena were poised to publish new findings that would describe in the most graphic terms yet the impact and costs of the global doctor deficit—and the tremendous potential to save lives.

In a report called *Essential Surgery*, the group calculated that if health-care systems in low-income countries had staff to perform just forty-four essential surgeries, they could save 1.5 million lives a year. Among the forty-four surgeries were burr holes and the VP shunts for hydrocephalus procedures that Dilan had taught Mayegga in Haydom.

The report also examined the economic contagion created by the surgical deficit—the challenges of affordability and transportation that people like the pregnant woman in the basket and her family experienced that day in Tanzania. Taking such factors into account, the group revealed that five billion people across the globe lack access to safe and affordable surgical care and anesthesia. Every year, more than 32.8 million people suffered ruinous expenditures related to conditions that could be treated with surgery. The report noted that without an urgent move to increase the world's surgical capacity, low- and middle-income countries would lose $12.3 trillion in productivity between 2015 and 2030.

The Ebola epidemic in Africa eventually was stopped. Many foreign doctors and nurses pulled out during the epidemic's early stages, but after West Africa's *ohayoda*, humanitarian groups and governments stood together; they sent troops to build tent hospitals; waves of doctors and nurses flowed into West Africa; groups such as Médecins Sans Frontières (Doctors Without Borders) worked heroically.

Sierra Leone lost nearly four thousand people to Ebola, but researchers in 2015 said that as many as 1.5 million people in that country needed some form of immediate surgery. The country has ten surgeons to heal these people. Except for a relatively small number of global health leaders, there has been no outcry about the surgical shortage, as there was for malaria, AIDS, Ebola, or the Zika virus. Until there is, from Tanzania to Honduras, people will die because someone like Mayegga couldn't treat their head wounds, someone like Nuwas couldn't repair their hernias, someone like Hayte couldn't perform cesarean sections. Millions of lives could be lost. Will there be an *ohayoda* for them?

ACKNOWLEDGMENTS
_____

In early 2010 Bill Hawkins, then executive editor of the *Post and Courier* in Charleston, told me, "I met this crazy brain surgeon who opened a guy's head with a wire saw in Africa. Check him out. Maybe we'll send you to Tanzania." Not many reporters get such an invitation, but thanks to Bill, I was soon on my way.

I owe an enormous debt of gratitude to the many Tanzanians I met on that and other trips, including Emmanuel Mighay, Anderson Sakweli, Clement Paresso, Emanuely Diyamay, Ibrahim Nyangura, and Innocent Shayo. Special thanks to Herman Malleyeck, who helped me understand Datoga culture. I spent many nights at Mama Naman's restaurant, partly for research purposes but mainly because there truly is something special about Naftali Naman and his wife, Haika.

I'm deeply thankful to the hospital's dedicated European staff, including Theresa Harbaurer, Jonas Rosenstok, Oystein Olsen, Mama Kari Olsen, and Olav and Turid Espegren, along with the many brilliant medical students and nurses I met in the dining hall.

Huge thanks also to former Tanzanian president Jakaya Kikwete, Mohamed Janabi, Haile Debas, Jennifer Edwards, Paul Young, Jonah Attebery, Rachel Chard, Joyce Nicholas, Pat Patten, Liesbeth Hoek, Maarten Hoek, Elizabeth Molyneux, D and Jane Word, Kathleen Ellis, Brennan Wesley, Sunil Patel, Robert Hamilton, Jim Kenning, Diane and Leonard Rodwell, Arthur Day, and Shannon Frazier for their thoughts and insights.

While reporting this story for the *Post and Courier*, I had the great fortune to receive a Harvard Nieman Fellowship. Thanks go to Bob Giles, Nieman curator at that time; Caroline Elkins, Harvard professor of history and African and African American studies; Paul Farmer; and Rose Moss, a wonderful writing instructor. All my Nieman friends were supportive, but special thanks to J. S. Tissainayagam, Darcy Frey, and Nazila Fathi, as well as to Antigone Barton, who read a late draft and provided invaluable corrections and insights. Thanks also to Mark Kessler, Katrin Hodapp, Laura Mamelok, Julia Wagner, and the rest of the Susanna Lea Associates team. In Canada, Brad Wilson was an early champion of the book, and Meg Masters, a remarkable editor who removed fatty tissue and tumors that likely would have killed the patient. In the United States, thanks to Helene Atwan, director of Beacon Press, for her passion about this complex story and to Andrea Lee for her careful copyediting.

This book wouldn't have happened without the support of the *Post and Courier*. Special thanks to Doug Pardue, a Pulitzer Prize–winning journalist who edited the original series. Thanks also to James Scott, a former P&C colleague and now a celebrated historian, and Bill Steiger of the *Physician Leadership Journal*.

The Fund for Investigative Journalism provided a pivotal travel grant. I'm honored to be among its beneficiaries.

It was my great honor to tell the stories of the three Tanzanian doctors featured in this book. Hayte Samo and I spent six hours talking one day in Dar es Salaam, a conversation about medicine and life I will never forget; Emanuel Nuwas is a sensitive and strong leader who has already proven to be a wonderful Tanzanian "Next Dr. Olsen."

And, I am particularly grateful to Emmanuel Mayegga, his wife, Samwayma, and their children, the 3Gs—Godwin, Glory, and Godlisten. Mayegga is a generous and complex man who opened his life and home to me because he believed his story would help others. He is a true doctor.

Perhaps the greatest privilege of all was learning about Carin and Dilan and their lovely family. Dilan's sisters, Vayomi and Hemali, provided important insights into their baby brother. Carin's brother and parents did the same for her. For a time I lived with Dilan's parents, Chitra and Somisara. Chitra fed me spectacular Sri

Lankan food and even more spectacular wisdom about body and mind. Sadly, Somisara passed away during the writing of this book. He had the spirit of a fighter and the soul of a teacher.

I'll be forever grateful to Carin and Dilan. They have a way of creating their own gravity. They taught me many things on this journey. They are heroic, brilliant, wonderfully flawed, generous, funny, honest, and altogether decent people devoted to making other people's lives healthier and happier, especially their beautiful children, Else, Dauwe, and Calla.

Finally, this book would not have happened without the support of my family, especially my mother, Margaret Bartelme, a public school teacher for more than four decades. Thanks and love go to Peter, Rachel, Nicki, David, and my son, Luke, who because of this book endured long absences even when I was home and sitting next to him. I am fortunate to have a life partner, Annie Duryee, who like Emmanuel Mayegga, used to walk around with a dictionary when she was a child. She read manuscripts of all shapes and sizes. She has my gratitude and love.

Several organizations support Haydom Lutheran Hospital, including Madaktari Africa (Madaktari.org), Friends of Haydom in Norway (www.haydom.no), and HaydomFriends of Germany (www.haydomfriends.de). Portions of the book's proceeds will be donated to groups such as these.

This book is based on hundreds of hours of interviews with Dilan and Carin Ellegala, Emmanuel Mayegga, Emanuel Nuwas, Hayte Samo, and the many other people whose lives fill these pages. Interviews were done in the United States and during five trips to Tanzania between 2010 and 2015. Other sources include academic journals, diaries, letters, medical records, and photographs.

I was present during many moments described in the book after 2010, when I first met Dilan. Since much of this story happens before that time, I've reconstructed scenes as best as fallible memories allow. When possible, I've confirmed dialogue with both participants. In some cases, particularly when Tanzanians spoke English for my benefit, I edited dialogue to capture the conversation's gist. To protect privacy of patients in both Tanzania and the United States, I changed some names and identifying details.

I witnessed numerous brain surgeries in Haydom and the United States, including Dilan's successful standstill in Lynchburg, Virginia. To build Mayegga's story, I spent many nights at Mama Naman's on the patio with him, at his home in Haydom, and in Dar es Salaam when he was in medical school. I noticed one night at Mama Naman's that he was staring at the horizon. "I always sit here so I can see where I came from," he told me.

Many books helped shape this one, including Charles Bosk, *Forgive and Remember: Managing Medical Failure* (1979); Michael Bliss, *Harvey Cushing: A Life in Surgery* (2005); David Eagleman, *Incognito:*

The Secret Lives of the Brain (2011); Bjorn Enes, *The Haydom Adventure* (2005); Suzanne Franks, *Reporting Disasters: Famine, Aid, Politics and the Media* (2013); and Atul Gawande, *Complications: A Surgeon's Notes on an Imperfect Science* (2002).

Also, John Iliffe's *Africans: The History of a Continent* (1995); Gerald Imber, *Genius on the Edge: The Bizarre Double Life of Dr. William Stewart Halsted* (2010); Robert Lupton, *Toxic Charity: How Churches and Charities Hurt Those They Help* (2011); Howard Markel, *An Anatomy of Addiction: Sigmund Freud, William Halsted, and the Miracle Drug Cocaine* (2011); George Monbiot, *No Man's Land: An Investigative Journey Through Kenya and Tanzania* (1994); Dambisa Moyo, *Dead Aid: Why Aid Is Not Working and How There Is a Better Way for Africa* (2009); and Jeffrey Sachs, *The End of Poverty: Economic Possibilities for Our Time* (2005).

Scientific and academic articles also were key sources, including Kristin D. Phillips, "Hunger, Healing, and Citizenship in Central Tanzania," *African Studies Review* (2009); Atul Gawande, "Two Hundred Years of Surgery," *New England Journal of Medicine* (2012); and Kurt Allen Ver Beek, "Lessons from the Sapling: Review of Quantitative Research on Short-Term Missions," in *Effective Engagement in Short-Term Missions*, ed. Robert J. Priest (2012).

Haile Debas's groundbreaking report in 2006 appeared in *Disease Control Priorities in Developing Countries*, 2nd ed., by the World Bank. Another thorough report is the Milbank Memorial Fund's *Health Worker Shortages and Global Justice* (2011), by Paula O'Brien and Lawrence O. Gostin.

Other important studies include Luke M. Funk et al., "Global Operating Theatre Distribution and Pulse Oximetry Supply," the *Lancet* (2010); Mark Shrime et al., "Charitable Platforms in Global Surgery: A Systematic Review of Their Effectiveness, Cost-Effectiveness, Sustainability, and Role Training," *World Journal of Surgery* (2015); John Meara et al., "Global Surgery 2030," the *Lancet* (2015); and *Essential Surgery*, vol. 1 of *Disease Control Priorities*, 3rd ed., World Bank Group.

·   ·   ·

Shannon Frazier did well after the standstill operation in Lynchburg. Eighteen months later, she told me: "I felt as if I was given a second chance at life."

A more extensive chapter-by-chapter breakdown of notes, references, citations, documents, and photos can be found at www.beacon.org/Bartelme.